# Neonatal, Adult and Paediatric Safe Transfer and Retrieval

## A Practical Approach to Transfers

# Neonatal, Adult and Paediatric Safe Transfer and Retrieval

## A Practical Approach to Transfers

Advanced Life Support Group

EDITED BY

Bernard Foëx

Peter-Marc Fortune

Cassie Lawn

**WILEY** Blackwell

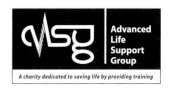

*Registered Offices*
John Wiley & Sons, Inc., 111 River Street, Hoboken, NJ 07030, USA
John Wiley & Sons Ltd, The Atrium, Southern Gate, Chichester, West Sussex, PO19 8SQ, UK

*Editorial Office*
9600 Garsington Road, Oxford, OX4 2DQ, UK

For details of our global editorial offices, customer services, and more information about Wiley products visit us at www.wiley.com.

Wiley also publishes its books in a variety of electronic formats and by print-on-demand. Some content that appears in standard print versions of this book may not be available in other formats.

A catalogue record for this book is available from the Library of Congress and the British Library

ISBN 9781119144922

Cover images: © BrianAJackson/Getty Images, © simonkr/Getty Images, © Mykhailo Lukashuk/Getty Images,
© Rawpixel.com/Shutterstock
Cover design by Wiley

Set in 10/12 pt Myriad Light by SPi Global, Pondicherry, India
Printed and bound in Singapore by Markono Print Media Pte Ltd

10  9  8  7  6  5  4  3  2  1

**Note to text:**
Drugs and their doses are mentioned in this text. Although every effort has been made to ensure accuracy, the writers, editors, publishers and printers cannot accept liability for errors or omissions. The final responsibility for delivery of the correct dose remains with the physician prescribing and administering the drug.

# Contents

# Working group

| | |
|---|---|
| **Bernard A. Foëx** | PhD, FRCSEd, FRCEM, FFICM, Consultant in Emergency Medicine and Critical Care, Manchester Royal Infirmary, Manchester University NHS Foundation Trust |
| **Simon Forrington** | FRCA, FFICM, Consultant Anaesthetics and Intensive Care Medicine, Manchester University NHS Foundation Trust |
| **Peter-Marc Fortune** | FRCPCH, FFICM, FAcadMEd, Consultant Paediatric Intensivist, Associate Medical Director, Royal Manchester Children's Hospital, Manchester |
| **Anneke Gyles** | MSc, BA Nursing, RN (Child), Advanced Nurse Practitioner, KIDS Intensive Care and Decision Support Service, Birmingham Women's and Children's Hospitals NHS Foundation Trust |
| **Steve Hancock** | FRCPCH, Consultant, Embrace Yorkshire and Humber Infant and Children's Transport Service |
| **Claire Harness** | RGN, RSCN, MSc, Deputy Director of Nursing, Sheffield Children's NHS Foundation Trust |
| **Carol Jackson** | MSc, BSc, RM, RN, Cheshire and Merseyside Neonatal Network Nurse Consultant for Neonatal Transport, Liverpool Women's NHS Foundation Trust, Liverpool Women's Hospital, Liverpool |
| **Peter Johnson** | Advanced Practitioner Critical Care, Royal Cornwall Hospital, Truro |
| **Cassie Lawn** | MB, BS, DRCOG, MRCGP, MRCPCH, Consultant Neonatologist, Royal Sussex County Hospital, Brighton |
| **Will Marriage** | Clinical Lead, Wales and West Acute Transport for Children |
| **Kate Parkins** | MRCPI (Paeds), FRCPCH, Consultant Paediatric Intensivist, Lead Consultant North West (England) and North Wales Paediatric Transport Service (NWTS) |
| **Thierry Spichiger** | Paramedic, Ambulance Service/ES ASUR, Vocational Training College for Registered Paramedics and Emergency Care, Switzerland |
| **Sue Wieteska** | CEO, Advanced Life Support Group, Manchester |

# Contributors

**Catherine Docherty** FRCA, PGCERT Medical Education, Consultant Paediatric Anaesthetist, Royal Manchester Children's Hospital, Manchester

**Mike Entwistle** MBBS, FRCA, FFICM, Consultant in Anaesthesia, Intensive Care and Transport Medicine, Royal Lancaster Infirmary and North West and North Wales Paediatric Transport Service (NWTS)

**Bernard A. Foëx** PhD, FRCSEd, FRCEM, FFICM, Consultant in Emergency Medicine and Critical Care, Manchester Royal Infirmary, Manchester University NHS Foundation Trust

**Simon Forrington** FRCA, FFICM, Consultant Anaesthetics and Intensive Care Medicine, Manchester University NHS Foundation Trust

**Peter-Marc Fortune** FRCPCH, FFICM, FAcadMEd, Consultant Paediatric Intensivist, Associate Medical Director, Royal Manchester Children's Hospital, Manchester

**Anneke Gyles** MSc, BA Nursing, RN (Child), Advanced Nurse Practitioner, KIDS Intensive Care and Decision Support Service, Birmingham Women's and Children's Hospitals NHS Foundation Trust

**Steve Hancock** FRCPCH, Consultant, Embrace Yorkshire and Humber Infant and Children's Transport Service

**Claire Harness** RGN, RSCN, MSc, Deputy Director of Nursing, Sheffield Children's NHS Foundation Trust

**Mark Hellaby** MSc, MEd, PG Cert, BSc (Hons), RODP, FHEA, North West Simulation Education Network Manager, NHS Health Education England

**Carol Jackson** MSc, BSc, RM, RN, Cheshire and Merseyside Neonatal Network Nurse Consultant for Neonatal Transport, Liverpool Women's NHS Foundation Trust, Liverpool Women's Hospital, Liverpool

**Peter Johnson** Advanced Practitioner Critical Care, Royal Cornwall Hospital, Truro

**Cassie Lawn** MB, BS, DRCOG, MRCGP, MRCPCH, Consultant Neonatologist, Royal Sussex County Hospital, Brighton

**Will Marriage** Clinical Lead, Wales and West Acute Transport for Children

**Graham Mason** MBChB, MRCPCH, Consultant Paediatric Critical Care, Royal Manchester Children's Hospital, Manchester University NHS Foundation Trust

**Kate Parkins** MRCPI (Paeds), FRCPCH, Consultant Paediatric Intensivist, Lead Consultant North West (England) and North Wales Paediatric Transport Service (NWTS)

# PaNSTaR (Paediatric and Neonatal Safe Transfer and Retrieval) first edition

## Working group

| | |
|---|---|
| **Peter Barry** | Paediatrics, Leicester |
| **Phil Booth** | Paediatrics, Aberdeen |
| **Steve Byrne** | Paediatrics/Neonatology, Middlesbrough |
| **Ian Dady** | Neonatology, Manchester |
| **Alan Fenton** | Neonatology, Newcastle |
| **Steve Fisher** | ALSG, Manchester |
| **Peter-Marc Fortune** | PICU, Manchester |
| **Claire Harness** | Neonatology, Leeds |
| **Carol Jackson** | Neonatal Transport, Liverpool |
| **Debbie Kenny** | University of Lancashire |
| **Cassie Lawn** | Neonatology, Brighton |
| **Andy Leslie** | Neonatology, Nottingham |
| **John Madar** | Neonatology, Plymouth |
| **Dawn McKimm** | Paediatric Transport Co-ordinator, Belfast |
| **Elaine Metcalfe** | ALSG, Manchester |
| **David Rowney** | Paediatric Anaesthesia and Intensive Care, Edinburgh |
| **Sue Wieteska** | ALSG, Manchester |

## Contributors

| | |
|---|---|
| **Steve Byrne** | Paediatrics/Neonatology, Middlesbrough |
| **Ian Dady** | Neonatology, Manchester |
| **Peter Driscoll** | Emergency Medicine, Manchester |
| **Peter-Marc Fortune** | PICU, Manchester |
| **Stephen Graham** | Anaesthetics, Middlesbrough |
| **Carol Jackson** | Neonatal Transport, Liverpool |
| **Cassie Lawn** | Neonatology, Brighton |
| **Daniel Lutman** | Children's Acute Transport Service, London |
| **Ian Macartney** | ICU, Manchester |
| **Kevin Mackway-Jones** | Emergency Medicine, Manchester |
| **John Madar** | Neonatology, Plymouth |
| **Dawn McKimm** | Paediatric Transport Co-ordinator, Belfast |

| | |
|---|---|
| **Mary Montgomery** | Children's Acute Transport Service, London |
| **Kate Parkins** | PICU, Liverpool |
| **Fiona Reynolds** | PICU, Birmingham |
| **Michael Tremlett** | Anaesthetics, Middlesbrough |
| **Allan Wardhaugh** | PICU, Cardiff |

# STaR (Safe Transfer and Retrieval) first and second editions

## Working group for first edition

| | |
|---|---|
| **Paul Allsop** | Anaesthetics, Burton-upon-Trent |
| **Paul Baines** | Paediatric ICU, Liverpool |
| **Ruth Buckley** | Emergency Nursing, Stoke on Trent |
| **John Burnside** | Ambulance Service, Manchester |
| **Peter Driscoll** | Emergency Medicine, Manchester |
| **Mark Forrest** | ICU, Liverpool |
| **Pauline Holt** | Paediatric ICU, Nursing, Liverpool |
| **Ian Macartney** | ICU, Manchester |
| **Kevin Mackway-Jones** | Emergency Medicine, Manchester |
| **Giles Morgan** | ICU, Portsmouth |
| **Peter Oakley** | Anaesthesia/Trauma, Stoke on Trent |
| **Claire O'Connor** | ICBIS Study, Manchester |
| **Vincent O'Keeffe** | ICU, Glan Clwyd |
| **Shirley Remington** | ICU, Manchester |
| **Stephen Shaw** | ICU, Liverpool |
| **Sarah Wheatly** | Anaesthesia, Manchester |
| **Susan Wieteska** | ALSG, Manchester |

## Working group for second edition

| | |
|---|---|
| **Peter Driscoll** | Emergency Medicine, Manchester |
| **Ian Macartney** | ICU, Manchester |
| **Kevin Mackway-Jones** | Emergency Medicine, Manchester |
| **Elaine Metcalfe** | ALSG, Manchester |
| **Giles Morgan** | ICU, Portsmouth |
| **Peter Oakley** | Anaesthesia/Trauma, Stoke on Trent |
| **Sarah Wheatly** | Anaesthesia, Manchester |
| **Susan Wieteska** | ALSG, Manchester |

## Contributors for second edition

| | |
|---|---|
| **Paul Allsop** | Anaesthetics, Burton-upon-Trent |
| **Paul Baines** | Paediatric ICU, Liverpool |
| **Danielle Bryden** | Anaesthesia, Manchester |

| | |
|---|---|
| **Ruth Buckley** | Emergency Nursing, Stoke on Trent |
| **John Burnside** | Ambulance Service, Manchester |
| **Jim Davies** | ICU, Merthyr Tydfil |
| **Peter Driscoll** | Emergency Medicine, Manchester |
| **Mark Forrest** | ICU, Liverpool |
| **Peter-Marc Fortune** | Paediatric ICU, Manchester |
| **Sarah Gill** | Emergency Nursing, Kilmarnock |
| **Tim Graham** | Cardiothoracic Surgery, Birmingham |
| **Colin Green** | Paediatrics, Folkestone |
| **Carl Gwinnutt** | Anaesthesia, Manchester |
| **Ann Hanson** | ICBIS, Manchester |
| **Pauline Holt** | Paediatric ICU Nursing, Liverpool |
| **Jonathan Hyde** | Cardiothoracic Surgery, West Midlands |
| **Peter Johnson** | ICU, Truro |
| **Ian Macartney** | ICU, Manchester |
| **Kevin Mackway-Jones** | Emergency Medicine, Manchester |
| **Elaine Metcalfe** | ALSG, Manchester |
| **Giles Morgan** | ICU, Portsmouth |
| **Peter Oakley** | Anaesthesia/Trauma, Stoke on Trent |
| **Claire O'Connor** | Formerly ICBIS Study, Manchester |
| **Vincent O'Keeffe** | ICU, Glan Clwyd |
| **Kate Olney** | ICBIS Study, Manchester |
| **Gillian Park** | Emergency Medicine, Harrow |
| **Shirley Remington** | ICU, Manchester |
| **Stephen Shaw** | ICU, Liverpool |
| **Gail Thomson** | Infectious Diseases, Manchester |
| **Terence Wardle** | Medicine, Chester |
| **Sarah Wheatly** | Anaesthesia, Manchester |
| **Susan Wieteska** | ALSG, Manchester |
| **Steve Wimbush** | ICU, Bristol |

# Preface

Transport medicine is recognised as a specialist area of clinical practice. It requires individuals to work safely and efficiently in small teams, often delivering very complex care in the mobile environment. For children there are only a small number of specialist centres able to deliver intensive care. This has led to the development of stand-alone transport services with teams solely dedicated to this work. For adults there is also a significant requirement to move unwell patients but the more evenly distributed specialist critical care services has led to a different model. Adult transport teams tend to be assembled from hospital personnel with additional training to work in the transport environment.

In addition to the critical care transfers, patients of all ages are often moved either within a hospital, or between hospitals in order to access diagnostic or therapeutic modalities that are not available locally. Although these movements may require much less technology and intensive support they are still subject to many of the same risks as transports of much sicker patients. These transfers are also generally carried out by staff who have not received training in transport medicine. This considerably raises the risk to the patient (and the staff), especially when the patient is approaching an acuity that might require critical care support.

Two courses and their manuals were developed to provide an introduction to the basic knowledge and principles needed to undertake the transfer of sick patients: Paediatric and Neonatal Safe Transfer and Retrieval (PaNSTaR) and (Adult) Safe Transfer and Retrieval (STaR). They were aimed both at those embarking on training in transport medicine and those who might expect to undertake such transfers on an occasional basis. Over the last few years it has become clear that some clinicians, particularly those based in district general hospitals, find themselves transferring both children and adults. Given that the principles of transport medicine are common across all age ranges it was decided to merge these two resources into one manual and one course: Neonatal, Adult and Paediatric Safe Transfer and Retrieval (NAPSTaR). This manual is the product of that fusion.

The focus is on inter-hospital transfers. However, the principles are also directly applicable every time a patient is moved between clinical areas. There are inevitably discussions of clinical situations throughout the text, however the focus is primarily on the logistics of the transfer process rather than the clinical detail. Those whose primary requirement is to enhance their knowledge of resuscitation should direct their reading to the Advanced Life Support (ALS), Advanced Paediatric Life Support (APLS), Advanced Resuscitation of the Newborn Infant (ARNI) and Newborn Life Support (NLS) manuals and courses as appropriate.

*Neonatal, Adult and Paediatric Safe Transfer and Retrieval: A Practical Approach to Transfers* has been developed by a multi-professional group from across the UK. A systematic approach is employed throughout that has its roots in both the original PaNSTaR and STaR courses.

The book is divided into six parts. Part 1 provides an introduction. Part 2 introduces the ACCEPT approach (see next page) and examines the component parts in detail. The practical issues that are encountered during the transfer process from an equipment perspective, and from a clinical perspective, are discussed in Part 3. Part 4 focuses on clinical considerations beginning with a generic overview and then specifically focusing on neonatal, paediatric and adult practice. Part 5 discusses particular situations and provides additional background information that is required to plan for special circumstances. The appendices in Part 6 contain supporting information and provide sample checklists and examples of documentation for those undertaking transfers.

Bernard Foëx, Peter-Marc Fortune and Cassie Lawn
Co-chairs NAPSTaR Working Group, 2019

| ACCEPT and SCRUMP principles | | |
|---|---|---|
| **Assessment** | **S Shared assessment** | What is the problem? (think summary)<br>What is being done? (think background)<br>What is the effect? (think assessment)<br>What is needed now? (think recommendation) |
| **Control** | | Identify team leader(s)<br>• Clinical<br>• Logistic<br>Identify and allocate tasks to be carried out<br>Pre-transport advice: ABCDEF |
| **Communication** | | Communication – what:<br>• Who you are – contact details<br>• What the problem is (soundbite)<br>• Relevant details<br>• What you need from the listener<br>• What you have done<br>• Effect of these actions<br>• Summarise agreed plans<br>• What you need from the listener    Communication – with who:<br>• Local team<br>• Transfer team<br>• Receiving team<br>• Ambulance control<br>• Family |
| **Evaluation** | | Establish urgency of transfer<br>Is the transfer appropriate – going to the right place?<br>Speed and mode of transfer |
| **Preparation Packaging** | **C Clinical isolation**<br>**R Resource limitation**<br>**U Unfamiliar equipment**<br>**M Movement and safety**<br>**P Physical/physiological changes)** | Checks of patient, equipment and personnel |
| **Transportation** | | Handover – CLEAR |

# Acknowledgements

A great many people have worked hard to produce this book and the accompanying course. The editors would like to thank all the contributors for their efforts and all NAPSTaR (formerly PaNSTaR and STaR) providers and instructors who took the time to send their comments during the development of the text and the course.

The NAPSTaR working group would like to acknowledge that this book has been developed from the preceding manuals and that a number of chapters in this book are essentially updates of those found in *Paediatric and Neonatal Safe Transfer and Retrieval: The Practical Approach* and *Safe Transfer and Retrieval: The Practical Approach* (second edition).

We thank the Difficult Airway Society (DAS), Great Ormond Street Hospital, National Tracheostomy Safety Project (NTSP) and North West and North Wales Paediatric Transport Service (NWTS) for the shared use of some of their figures and algorithms. We also thank Kathryn Claydon-Smith, Joanne Cooke, Brendan McGrath, Richard Neal, Matthew Davis, Paul Reavley and Mark Woolcock for sharing their photographs and illustrations.

Finally, we would like to thank, in advance, those of you who will attend the NAPSTaR course for your continued constructive comments regarding the future development of both the course and the manual.

# Contact details and website information

ALSG: www.alsg.org

For details on ALSG courses visit the website or contact:
Advanced Life Support Group
ALSG Centre for Training and Development
29–31 Ellesmere Street
Swinton, Manchester
M27 0LA
Tel: +44 (0)161 794 1999
Fax: +44 (0)161 794 9111
Email: enquiries@alsg.org

Clinicians practising in tropical and under-resourced healthcare systems are advised to read *International Maternal and Child Health Care – A Practical Manual for Hospitals Worldwide* (www.mcai.org.uk) which gives details of additional relevant illnesses not included in this text.

## Updates

The material contained within this book is updated on a 5-yearly cycle. However, practice may change in the interim period. We will post any changes on the ALSG website, so we advise that you visit the website regularly to check for updates (www.alsg.org).

## References

All references are available on the NAPSTaR course pages on the ALSG website www.alsg.org.

## On-line feedback

It is important to ALSG that the contact with our providers continues after a course is completed. We now contact everyone 6 months after their course has taken place asking for on-line feedback on the course. This information is then used whenever the course is updated to ensure that the course provides optimum training to its participants.

# How to use your textbook

## The anytime, anywhere textbook

**Wiley E-Text**

Your textbook comes with free access to a **Wiley E-Text: Powered by VitalSource** version – a digital, interactive version of this textbook which you own as soon as you download it.

Your **Wiley E-Text** allows you to:

**Search:** Save time by finding terms and topics instantly in your book, your notes, even your whole library (once you've downloaded more textbooks)
**Note and Highlight:** Colour code, highlight and make digital notes right in the text so you can find them quickly and easily
**Organise:** Keep books, notes and class materials organised in folders inside the application
**Share:** Exchange notes and highlights with friends, classmates and study groups
**Upgrade:** Your textbook can be transferred when you need to change or upgrade computers
**Link:** Link directly from the page of your interactive textbook to all of the material contained on the companion website

The **Wiley E-Text** version will also allow you to copy and paste any photograph or illustration into assignments, presentations and your own notes.

### *To access your Wiley E-Text:*

- Find the redemption code on the inside front cover of this book and carefully scratch away the top coating of the label.
- Go to https://online.vitalsource.co.uk and log in or create an account. Go to Redeem and enter your redemption code to add this book to your library.
- Or to download the Bookshelf application to your computer, tablet or mobile device go to www.vitalsource.com/software/bookshelf/downloads.
- Open the Bookshelf application on your computer and register for an account.
- Follow the registration process and enter your redemption code to download your digital book.
- If you have purchased this title as an e-book, access to your **Wiley E-Text** is available with proof of purchase within 90 days. Visit http://support.wiley.com to request a redemption code via the 'Live Chat' or 'Ask A Question' tabs.

---

**The VitalSource Bookshelf can now be used to view your Wiley E-Text on iOS, Android and Kindle Fire!**

- **For iOS:** Visit the app store to download the VitalSource Bookshelf: http://bit.ly/17ib3XS
- **For Android and Kindle Fire:** Visit the Google Play Market to download the VitalSource Bookshelf: http://bit.ly/BSAAGP

You can now sign in with the email address and password you used when you created your VitalSource Bookshelf Account.
Full E-Text support for mobile devices is available at: http://support.vitalsource.com

---

We hope you enjoy using your new textbook. Good luck with your studies!

# PART 1
# Introduction

# CHAPTER 1
# Introduction

## Learning outcomes

After reading this chapter, you will be able to:
- Describe why unwell patients are transferred between hospitals
- Identify the issues that may adversely affect delivery of care

## 1.1 Background

In children's critical care alone there are in excess of 5000 paediatric intensive care unit (PICU) transfers between hospitals and 16 000 transfers of neonatal patients in the UK every year. In addition to this there are numerous high dependency unit (HDU) and non-urgent transfers between centres and countless thousands of intra-hospital transfers undertaken by healthcare professionals every year. Each one of these transfers represents an episode of care which is associated with a period of increased risk for both the child and the clinical staff. These risks can at best be eliminated and at the least be minimised through appropriate training.

The NAPSTaR manual together with its associated course is aimed at a multi-disciplinary audience and has been developed to provide a comprehensive introduction and overview of the process of transferring unwell patients. Its conception followed from the success of the PaNSTaR and STaR manuals and courses. The underpinning concepts described herein, and in particular the ACCEPT principles, are essentially the same.

Throughout the text the use of the words 'child' or 'children' should be taken to refer to the entire age range (neonate up to 16 years of age). Where appropriate, more specific references to particular age groups will be made where practices vary according to age. Neonates will be used to refer to all preterm babies and also term babies of less than 28 days of age. Infants shall refer to all those under 1 year and adults for those over 18 years. Parent refers to any person with parental responsibility.

With regard to the transfer of children there has been a cultural change which has occurred in many centres where non-paediatricians have distanced themselves from paediatric practice, triggered by the centralisation of paediatric services. Many district general hospital (DGH) practitioners, faced with a critically ill child, may now find themselves practicing at the edge of their comfort zone. This is perhaps particularly true if they have to undertake a transfer.

Most neonatal intensive care units (NICUs) and PICUs will have an associated retrieval team. However, the majority, if not all, of these teams are not sufficiently resourced to be able to provide a robust service 100% of the time.

In adult practice most centres do not have a dedicated transport team and transfer teams are drawn from in-patient staff (often from critical care). There will be occasions, such as patients with surgically treatable lesions following a traumatic head injury, where current practice would dictate that the referring hospital should undertake the transfer in order to minimise the time to neurosurgery. These factors mean that referring centres may expect to carry out the transfer for up to 25% of the children that they refer for urgent tertiary care.

*Neonatal, Adult and Paediatric Safe Transfer and Retrieval: A Practical Approach to Transfers*, First Edition.
Edited by Bernard Foëx, Peter-Marc Fortune and Cassie Lawn.
© 2019 John Wiley & Sons Ltd. Published 2019 by John Wiley & Sons Ltd.

Reading this manual and attending a NAPSTaR course will provide you with the basic strategies and background that you need to join a transfer team. It is important to note that proficiency in this area only comes with the additional training and experience that may be gained from working with practitioners already experienced in this area.

## 1.2 The approach to transfer

Any transfer process may be broken down into three components:

- Organisational and management strategy
- Practical issues
- Training required to appropriately use the equipment needed during the transfer

The course focus is on the transportation of patients between hospitals. However, the same approach can, and should, be applied to the transportation of unwell patients within hospitals.

The usual purpose of an inter-hospital transfer or retrieval is either to allow the patient to be treated more effectively or to obtain additional diagnostic information, in a geographically separate site. Transfer per se does not constitute therapy and represents a time of increased risk. It is therefore essential to always consider the risks versus the benefits before undertaking a potentially hazardous journey.

In the neonatal population, babies may be transferred acutely because they require intensive care unit (ICU) therapy that is not available at the referring hospital. There are also a significant number of neonates that may be moved for specialist examinations or opinions. Infants and older children are primarily transferred when they are acutely unwell to a central PICU or HDU. Some transfers will also occur for secondary or tertiary opinions, but the majority of these patients will not present a clinical risk and will be transported by their parents. In acute cases, children may sometimes have to be transferred significant distances, especially at busy times such as midwinter, as beds may not be available in their nearest tertiary centre.

The source of patients also varies widely:

- Delivery suite
- Emergency department
- NICU
- Adult ICU
- Paediatric wards
- Theatres
- HDU
- Coronary care unit

Emergency departments are probably the most frequent starting places for the movement of PICU patients. Sometimes children are moved to local critical care facilities prior to transfer. Either way, the adequacy of resuscitation and the degree of packaging that will have been undertaken before the arrival of the transfer team is highly variable. When dispatching a team to undertake a transfer it is always best to assume they will need to do everything and therefore must have the knowledge and skills to do this.

Transfers are not infrequently associated with adverse events, which may be recorded on transfer forms. Those seen most commonly are:

- Supply failure (electrical power, gases, fluids or drugs)
- Equipment failure
- Significant hypotension
- Significant hypoxia
- Inadequate resuscitation
- Significant tachycardia
- Mechanical ventilator not available
- No capnography available (when clinically indicated)
- Delay in getting ambulance
- Ambulance getting lost en route
- Cardiac arrest in ambulance

The number of inter-hospital transfers continues to rise. This is perhaps driven by increasing expectations on the part of both the public and healthcare professionals.

This manual will provide those who may be involved with the transfer of unwell patients with a systematic approach to guide their work. It does not seek to teach or develop the clinical skills required to undertake such care but it does provide a structure that should help eliminate the majority of the non-clinical pitfalls. There is no substitute for the practical training that may be gained by working with those experienced in this field.

# CHAPTER 2
# Medicine on the move

## Learning outcomes

After reading this chapter, you will be able to:
- Describe how transport medicine differs from hospital-based care
- State key themes that must be considered before moving a patient

## 2.1 Introduction

Moving patients from one clinical environment to another is a process that requires careful thought, preparation and attention to detail. This move could be from a home environment to hospital, from the scene of an accident to an emergency department, from a hospital ward to a computed tomography (CT) or magnetic resonance imaging (MRI) scanner or from one hospital to another. In any scenario, it is essential that the staff involved in moving the patient have given due consideration to the process of the move, considered what equipment and monitoring is required, who should accompany the patient and the best means of transport.

## 2.2 SCRUMP

This chapter aims to briefly outline some of the considerations that come to bear at the time any transport is initiated. These issues will be dealt with in more detail later in the manual, but can be usefully brought to mind using the acronym **SCRUMP**.

**SCRUMP**

**S**  Shared assessment
**C**  Clinical isolation
**R**  Resource limitation
**U**  Unfamiliar equipment
**M**  Movement and safety
**P**  Physical and physiological changes

### Shared assessment

Whenever a patient is to be moved from one environment to another, the teams must share key information about the patient's clinical condition. The subsequent decision making is based on these shared assessments. For example, a neurosurgeon may advise that a patient is transferred as quickly as possible; a radiographer may suggest that a patient is brought to the scanner immediately; an intensive care unit may suggest that it is safe for a patient to remain locally for a number of hours before they are transferred: the team leader needs to assimilate all information and recommendations and agree a plan with the multi-disciplinary teams This will ensure that each transport episode can be undertaken safely.

### Clinical isolation

Whenever a patient is moved from one location to another, they are at their most vulnerable during the physical transit. For example, transferring from a bed to stretcher, moving within a building or moving from one building to another. In addition the team may be physically separated from their usual support structures. It is essential that everything possible

*Neonatal, Adult and Paediatric Safe Transfer and Retrieval: A Practical Approach to Transfers*, First Edition.
Edited by Bernard Foëx, Peter-Marc Fortune and Cassie Lawn.
© 2019 John Wiley & Sons Ltd. Published 2019 by John Wiley & Sons Ltd.

is done to minimise the risks and to optimise care during any period of isolation. There are numerous strategies to reduce the risks such as structured competency-based training; the use of local expertise and resources; clear protocols; and documentation. Structured support can be achieved through telephone communications or other channels, or in person, or even by dispatching senior help when necessary.

### Resource limitation

Unlike working in a hospital environment, transport clinicians are limited by what they have chosen to take with them, what they are physically able to carry and by their ability to access this kit in the transport environment. Inevitably, all equipment and supplies will be carried in limited quantities, but the most common transport incidents are caused by loss of gas supply, loss of electrical power and by vehicular failure (including running out of fuel!). Planning and preparation will allow transport clinicians to estimate the consumables required during the transfer in order to minimise the risk of such events.

### Unfamiliar equipment

The equipment that is used in the transport environment is often different from that in use within a hospital setting. Monitors, saturation probes, syringe drivers and ventilators will all be chosen for their transport characteristics and may be less sophisticated than their hospital-based counterparts. It is essential that all those involved in transporting patients are not only able to use the equipment safely but can troubleshoot devices if they do not operate in the expected manner. A system of equipment competency-based training is essential to ensure that patient safety is maintained during transport.

### Movement and safety

Physically moving any patient confers specific risks. For example, in intra-hospital transfers, the main risks are displacement of tubes, catheters and lines, and equipment failure. Inter-hospital transfer carries added risks. UK accident data show several hundred incidents involving ambulances each year, frequently resulting in serious injury and occasionally in fatalities. These facts lead to many specific considerations – how the patient is best secured to their trolley; how equipment, pumps and monitors are safely secured; how staff members are seated and strapped when in a moving vehicle; and the speed and driving characteristics of any journey.

### Physical and physiological changes

The cramped, noisy, vibrating and poorly lit environment of an ambulance or aircraft cabin provides specific challenges to any team moving a patient, as does movement within and between buildings and vehicles. Issues include thermoregulation, where there may be a conflict between a desire to keep a patient under close observation versus the need to keep them warm; the ability to see and hear monitors and alarms, where line of sight may be restricted and there are competing sounds and noises; issues surrounding acceleration and deceleration; and the whole area of altitude physiology for flight transfers.

Each of these aspects of care will be dealt with more fully in Chapter 11.

SCRUMP provides an overview of the differences and challenges of transport medicine when compared with static hospital care.

## 2.3 ACCEPT

The NAPSTaR structure for the practical delivery of safe patient transfer is captured through the **ACCEPT** principles.

---

**ACCEPT**

**A**   Assessment
**C**   Control
**C**   Communication
**E**   Evaluation
**P**   Preparation and packaging
**T**   Transportation

---

These will be discussed in detail throughout this text with reference to the challenges of medicine on the move identified by SCRUMP.

# CHAPTER 3
# Planning the move

## Learning outcomes

After reading this chapter, you will be able to:
- Define the complexity of transfer planning
- Name the factors that should be considered when planning a transfer
- Prepare for the likely events during transfer
- Recognise the need to appropriately plan for the worst case scenario

## 3.1 Introduction

The decision to move a patient pivots on a number of factors. The requirement for transfer may be to an internal location, such as the computed tomography (CT) scanner or theatres, or external, to another centre with staffing of facilities not available on the current site. The decision to proceed and the timing of the transfer must be based on balancing the benefits of the transfer against the clinical risk posed to the patient and team by the transfer. Whilst on most occasions this can be quite straightforward, there are a significant number of occasions where the risk of deterioration or even death en route will need to be weighed up in this analysis.

The first stage of this process is to gather all the key information required. This will usually be achieved during the assessment stage of the process but further information may also be needed.

The following information should be considered as a minimum dataset.

**Patient**
- Clinical assessment of the patient's status:
  - How stable is the patient? (**ABCDEF** approach)
  - If unstable, is it possible to stabilise and how long might that be expected to take?
- An assessment of the likelihood of deterioration during transfer based on:
  - Diagnosis (if known)
  - Current status and physiological trends
  - Need to transfer before optimal stabilisation
  - Specific condition/transport factors, e.g.
    - Severe pulmonary dysfunction and air travel
    - Mobile extracorporeal membrane oxygenation
- Rationale for transfer, e.g. access to specialist care

**Staff and logistics**
- Staff:
  - Availability of staff with suitable competencies
  - Risk of removing expert staff from local unit (if local transfer team)
- Expected time taken for transfer (impacts on above)
- Safety of the transfer – weather/mode of transfer

---

**ABCDEF approach**

**A**  Airway assessment and control
**B**  Breathing
**C**  Circulation
**D**  Disability
**E**  Exposure (including temperature in neonates and children) and everything else
**F**  Family

---

## 3.2  Patient risk assessment

Increasingly, patient track and trigger systems (or early warning systems (EWS)) are embedded in hospital practice and are a tool for identifying patient deterioration by analysing physiological parameters. The monitored physiological parameters are scored, and when a threshold abnormal score is reached a clinical review is triggered.

The EWS may be employed in conjunction with a structured ABCDEF assessment to help highlight specific clinical risks associated with transport. The likelihood of deterioration during transfer may be assessed through serial EWS and reassessments of ABCDEF. An understanding of the progression of the disease process together with the likelihood of requiring additional interventions during transportation and an understanding of the clinical benefit of transfer will inform when to move a patient.

It is important to recognise both the advantages and limitations of EWS. They are designed to provide an alert, usually on the general wards, when a patient is likely to be unwell or deteriorating. It is critical to understand that a low score should never be used to provide reassurance when there are other worrying factors in the clinical assessment. It is also true that EWS are relatively insensitive to ongoing deterioration once a patient is decompensating and has already generated a high score. In summary, EWS are a useful adjunct to structured clinical assessment, which should always be the primary assessment tool. The patient's lead consultant should always be contacted if at any time there is any doubt about this assessment. They in turn may choose to discuss the patient's status with other colleagues or experts at the receiving centre where appropriate.

## 3.3  Staff and logistics risk assessment

Patient assessment for transfer should always be viewed in the context of the duration and mode of transport. The longer a transfer the more time there is for deterioration to occur. Even short transfers, within a hospital, may not be without challenges. For example, when going outside, between buildings, or when utilising a lift, never go without supplies for at least 30 minutes!

When travelling between centres the mode of transport may also present specific risks. In all cases there will be some limitation of access to the patient and equipment, and the team may not be 100% familiar with the environment and may have to cope with complex logistics. The latter is especially true for air transfers where there are also the effects of altitude physiology to consider.

The staff accompanying a patient must have suitable competencies to deliver clinical care not only at the current level of dependency of the patient, but also at an increased dependency level in the event of deterioration. In an ideal world, staff should neither be fatigued nor stressed and they should always be familiar with all the transport equipment, policies and procedures (see Chapter 4).

Adverse weather conditions such as snow, ice or poor visibility should always be factored into the assessment of the need for transfer. Risks of this type can be reduced by using familiar vehicles and modes of transport, by altering routes or delaying the transfer; an alternative destination may need to be considered for very long transfers. The use of sirens and blue lights to facilitate anything more than progression at safe, standard road speeds should be avoided wherever possible. High speed transfers have no impact on clinical outcome, but expose the patient, the team and the public to considerably enhanced risk. Safety of the team and patient is the absolute priority.

## 3.4  Use of physiological measurements in identifying transfer risk

The clinical risk of the transfer and the level of competence required by escorting staff will be informed by the patient's condition. As discussed previously, a physiological track and trigger system (EWS) may, under certain circumstances, be used in combination with other parameters ($SpO_2$, Glasgow Coma Scale (GCS), base excess) to risk assess patients prior to transfer.

For the purposes of discussion, the risk may be divided into categories of low, medium and high. The EWS score may be used to inform this classification but will be dependent on the score used and therefore must be calibrated locally.

### Low risk group

This group includes all patients with near normal physiology. In this group there are no additional concerns and these patients should have a low risk of clinical deterioration during transfer, although some clinical competences may be required during transfer, e.g. oxygen therapy or infusion therapy.

### Medium risk group

These patients will have clear evidence of systemic illness or instability. They are likely to have an EWS score in the middle of the range. The group may include patients who would fit the criteria for high dependency care.

This group are potentially the highest risk transfers. They may be transported with the minimum of technological support but could be of risk of major deterioration during transfer. They require a detailed pre-transfer assessment that should be based on an ABCDEF approach. The following should be considered:

- Is the general condition of the patient improving, stable or deteriorating?
- Review the rationale for the transfer:
  - Does the need/benefit for investigation or enhanced support outweigh the transfer risks?
  - Is this the right time to transfer?
- How long will the transfer take?
- What physiological deterioration may occur during the transfer?
- What competences are required during the transfer?

If after making the assessment, there are concerns for the patient's safety during transfer, these must be discussed with senior medical staff. If it is judged appropriate to proceed, it is vital that the transfer team have the competencies to cope with the very worst case scenario. It is neither safe nor fair to the patient or staff to compromise on this.

### High risk group

Patients in this group will have significant physiological derangement or have a condition that would be expected to rapidly deteriorate during transfer. They will usually have already have triggered an emergency response from the critical care team. A formal risk assessment and consideration of the cause, as described for the medium risk patient, must be undertaken.

Patients in this group must only be transferred by a team with critical care competencies.

## 3.5 Categories of transfer

It is possible to spend a great deal of time categorising the types and subtypes of patient transfers. However, for practical purposes they can be divided into the following categories, which will be considered separately below. The terminology used differs slightly between adult and paediatric/neonatal practice; where this is the case the neonatal categories are shown in **bold**.

- Major trauma
- Emergency
  - unstable (*Time critical*) (**Time critical**)
  - stable (*Intensive*) (**Uplift of care**)
- Urgent (ill and stable) (**Capacity transfer**)
- Elective (planned) (**Repatriation**)

### Major trauma

This category effectively sits in parallel to the emergency and urgent/unstable categories. The clinical priorities and management are almost identical to those for medical and non-trauma surgical emergency patients, but it is separated out because separate protocols and infrastructures exist to manage these patients within trauma networks.

- All major trauma transfers must be discussed with the local major trauma centre
- Every patient should arrive at the major trauma centre within 3 hours (if urban) or within 4 hours (if rural) of injury

- Patients should always be transferred with minimum delay once they have a secure airway and have secure IV access. Transfer should NOT be delayed for investigations such as CT scans
- Ongoing vigilance and, where appropriate, stabilisation during the transfer is required to avoid secondary injury

### Emergency

Time critical transfers are prompted by the clinical need for the patient to receive life- or limb-saving interventions that are not available in the referring centre. Examples of such scenarios include acute neurological, non-traumatic, space-occupying lesions or patients requiring advanced respiratory therapy such as high frequency oscillation.

- Communication is key, allowing for advice in patient management from the receiving hospital/unit. This in turn allows the local transfer team more time to focus on patient management
- The patient should be transferred without delay once they have an appropriately secured airway and IV access
- Careful consideration should be given to delaying the transfer in order to place arterial or central lines. If in doubt such decisions should be discussed with the lead consultant and the leads in the transfer and receiving teams
- Ongoing vigilance and appropriate stabilisation during transfer will be required to maintain the patient in the best possible physiological condition
- Transfer may need to be undertaken by local staff ('ad hoc transport team') to avoid delay. This requirement may require some pragmatic decision making by the leads in the referring, transferring and receiving services

### Urgent

These patients require urgent transfer for ongoing care, they may be requiring intensive, high dependency or lesser levels of care and may be stable or unstable. The time spent locally preparing a patient for transfer depends very much on the risk assessment process described earlier.

- Many emergency transfers require intensive care delivered by an appropriately trained team
- Communication with the receiving unit is key
- Placement of arterial lines, central lines, etc. should usually be undertaken prior to transfer
- Ongoing stabilisation during transfer may to be required to avoid secondary injury, but wherever possible should be the exception rather than the rule

### Elective

These patients are often moved within or between hospitals for specialist care or investigations. The timing of the transfer is dependent on the risk assessment as described. A typical example of this would be a neonatal patient requiring therapy for retinopathy of prematurity.

## 3.6 Summary

The decision to commit to and execute the transfer of a patient depends on a balanced risk assessment. All of the risks associated with the transfer posed by the physical movement, limitations on treatment, logistics and the physical safety of the patient, staff and public should be considered. A clinician with appropriate experience and seniority must always be involved with this process.

The transfer team must always have the competencies to cope with the worst possible scenarios that could develop during transfer. In time critical situations, a degree of pragmatism is required in this regard where significant injury or death is likely without the transfer.

# CHAPTER 4
# Human factors

---

### Learning outcomes

After reading this chapter, you will be able to:
- Describe how human factors affect the performance of individuals and teams in the healthcare environment

---

## 4.1 Introduction

The management of emergency care has traditionally concentrated on knowledge of the treatment process. This might be, for example, when to give a specific intervention, drug or fluid aliquot. An often overlooked element is how in these high pressure situations individuals from a variety of different professional and specialty backgrounds come together to form an effective team that minimises errors and works actively to prevent adverse events.

This chapter provides a brief introduction to some of the human factors that can affect the performance of individuals and teams in the complex healthcare environment. Human factors, also sometimes referred to as ergonomics, is an established scientific discipline and clinical human factors has been described as:

> *Enhancing clinical performance through an understanding of the effects of teamwork, tasks, equipment, workspace, culture and organisation on human behaviour and abilities and application of that knowledge in clinical settings.*

## 4.2 Extent of healthcare error

In 2000 an influential report entitled *To Err is Human: Building a Safer Health System* suggested that across the USA somewhere between 44 000 and 98 000 deaths each year could be attributed to medical error. A pilot study in the UK demonstrated that approximately one in 10 patients admitted for healthcare experienced an adverse event.

Healthcare has been able to learn from a number of other high risk industries including the nuclear, petrochemical, space exploration, military and aviation industries about how team issues have been managed. These lessons have been slowly adopted and translated to healthcare.

Specialist working groups and national bodies have been instrumental in promoting awareness of the importance of human factors in healthcare. They aim to raise awareness and promote the principles and practices of human factors, to identify current human factor activity, capability and barriers and to create conditions to support human factors being embedded at a local level. One such example of this is the UK Clinical Human Factors Group and the National Quality Board's concordat statement on human factors.

## 4.3 Causes of healthcare error

Consider this example of an adverse event:

> A patient needs to receive an infusion of a particular drug. An error occurs and the patient receives an incorrect drug. What are the potential causes of this situation (Table 4.1)?

---

*Neonatal, Adult and Paediatric Safe Transfer and Retrieval: A Practical Approach to Transfers*, First Edition.
Edited by Bernard Foëx, Peter-Marc Fortune and Cassie Lawn.
© 2019 John Wiley & Sons Ltd. Published 2019 by John Wiley & Sons Ltd.

| **Table 4.1** Potential causes of our example drug error | |
|---|---|
| Prescription error | Wrong drug prescribed |
| Preparation error | Correct drug prescribed but misread |
| Preparation error | Contents mislabelled during manufacture |
| Drawing up error | Incorrect drug selected |
| Administration error | Patient ID mix-up leading to drug given to wrong patient |

Q. What one thing links all of these errors?

A. The humans involved – these are all examples of human errors.

Humans make mistakes. No amount of checks and procedures will mitigate this fact. In fact the only way to completely remove human errors is to remove all the humans involved. It is vital therefore that we look to work in a way that, wherever possible, minimises the occurrence of mistakes and ensures that when they do occur the chance of it resulting in an adverse event is also minimised.

## 4.4 Human error

It has been suggested that human errors can be further categorised into those that occur at the sharp end of care by the treating team and individuals and those at a blunt or organisational level, typically through policies, procedures, staffing and culture. These errors can be further subdivided (Table 4.2).

| **Table 4.2** Types of errors | | Explanation | Example |
|---|---|---|---|
| **Sharp errors that occur with the team/ individuals treating the patient** | Mistake | Lack or misapplication of knowledge | Not knowing the correct drug to prescribe |
| | Slip or lapse | Skills-based mistake | Knowing the correct drug but writing another one |
| | Violation | Deliberate action that may be routine or exceptional | Not attempting to get a drug second checked as staff are not available |
| **Blunt/organisational errors** | | Policies, procedures, infrastructure and building layout that has errors embedded | Different drugs used by different specialities and departments for same condition |

It is typically found that latent/organisational issues often coexist with sharp errors; in fact it is rare for an isolated error to occur, often there is a chain of events that results in the adverse event. The Swiss cheese model demonstrates how apparently random, unconnected events and organisational decisions can all make errors more likely (Figure 4.1). Conversely, a standardised system with good defences can capture these errors and prevent adverse events.

Each of the slices of Swiss cheese represents barriers which, under ideal circumstances, would prevent or detect the error. The holes represent weaknesses in these barriers; if the holes align the error passes through undetected.

Reconsider the example of drug error using the Swiss cheese model. The first slice is the doctor writing the prescription, the second slice is the organisation's drug policy, the third is the nurse who draws up the drug and the fourth is the nurse who second checks the drug.

Now consider the following. What if the doctor is very junior and not familiar with that area or those drugs? – that slice of cheese has larger holes. What if the organisation has failed to develop a robust drug policy that is fit for purpose? – this second slice is considerably weakened or may even be removed completely. What if the nurse is a bank nurse who does not normally work on this ward and is not familiar with commonly used drugs? – their slice has also got larger holes.

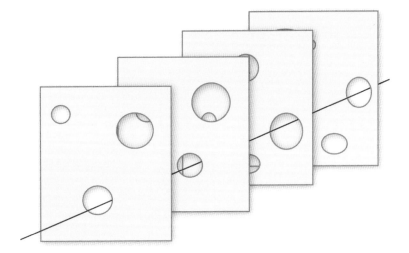

**Figure 4.1 The Swiss cheese model**

What if this area is always short of staff so staff do not routinely attempt to get the drug second checked? – this slice is completely removed.

The end result is that multiple defences have been weakened or removed and error is more likely, and the error is more likely to cause harm. Also be aware of the different types of error with potential gaps in knowledge, a latent/organisational error (no effective policy and possibly an issue with nurse staffing) and a routine violation.

## 4.5  Learning from error

Historically, those making mistakes have been identified and singled out for punishment and/or retraining, in what is often referred to as a culture of blame. With our example, drug error blame would most likely have fallen on the shoulders of the nurse administering and/or the doctor incorrectly prescribing. Does retraining these individuals make it safer for other or future patients? That clearly depends on the underlying reasons. If it was purely a knowledge gap, possibly, but does the same knowledge gap exist elsewhere? Potentially all the other issues remain unresolved. Moreover, such punitive reactions make it less likely for individuals to admit mistakes and near misses in future.

The focus is now on learning from error and is shifting away from the individual; learning is much more focused on determining the system/organisational errors. Ensuring there are robust systems, procedures and policies in place can reduce errors. Issues will still need to be addressed where individuals have been reckless or lacked knowledge – but consideration is now given to reasons why the individuals felt the need to violate or did not have access to the knowledge required.

For this approach to work health services need to learn from errors, adverse events and near misses. This requires engagement at both the individual level, by reporting errors, and the organisational level, investigating and feeding back the learning using a systematic approach. It is also key that learning is cascaded through the organisation and across the health service to raise awareness and prevent similar situations from recurring.

Violation may be indicative of the failure of systems, procedures or policies or other cultural issues. It is important that policies, procedures, roles and even buildings and equipment are all designed proactively with human factors in mind so things do not have to be fixed retrospectively when adverse events occur. This means that all members of the organisation must be aware of human factors, not just the front-line clinical staff.

### Improving team and individual performance

Having discussed the magnitude of the problem of healthcare error, the rest of this chapter will focus on how the team and individuals' performance can be developed.

Raising awareness of human factors and being able to practise these skills and behaviours within multi-professional teams allows the development of effective teams in all situations. Simulation activity allows a team to explore these new ideas, practise them and develop them. To do this we need feedback on our performance within a safe environment where no patient is at risk and egos and personal interests can be set aside. Consider how you developed a clinical skill. It was something that needed to be practised again and again until eventually it started to become automatic and routine. The same applies for our human factor behaviours. In addition, recognising our inherent human limitations and the situations when errors are more likely to occur will improve vigilance and reduce risk.

## 4.6 Communication

Lack of communication is the leading cause of adverse events. This is not surprising; to have an effective team there needs to be good communication. The leader needs to communicate with the followers, and followers communicate with leaders and other followers. Communication is not just saying something – it is ensuring that information is accurately passed on and received (Table 4.3). We all want to ensure effective communication at all times. Remember there are multiple components to effective communication.

**Table 4.3** Elements of communication

| Sender | Sender | Transmitted | Receiver | Receiver |
| --- | --- | --- | --- | --- |
| Thinks of what to say | Says message | Through air, over phone or via email | Hears it | Thinks about it and acts |

When communicating face to face a great deal of information is transmitted non-verbally, which can make telephone or email conversations more challenging. Communication can be more difficult when talking across professional, specialty or hierarchal barriers as we do not always talk the same technical language, have the same levels of understanding or even have a full awareness of the other person's role.

There are a variety of similar tools to aid communication such as SBAR (situation, background, assessment and recommendation). Find out what your organisation uses and practice using it; look out for other staff using it too. SBAR is designed for acute clinical communications. It helps the sender to plan and organise the message, make it succinct and focused, and provide it in a logical and expected order. It is also an empowerment tool allowing the sender (who may be more junior) to request an action from a more senior individual. While these tools are useful, they tend to be reserved for certain situations whereas we want to establish effective communication as the routine not the exception. One method to routinely improve communication is to incorporate a feedback loop.

### Effective communication with a feedback loop

Errors can occur at any level or multiple levels. Consider a busy clinical situation and the team leader shouts 'We need an ECG connecting' while looking at the blood pressure – what happens? The majority of times nothing – nobody goes to connect the ECG! So how can this be improved? Most obviously an individual can be identified to perform the task, by name: 'Michael can you please connect the ECG?' If Michael says 'yes' effective communication might be assumed; but not always. What has Michael heard and what will he do? At the moment we do not really know what message has been received. If Michael dashes over with a cup of tea, this is because 'Michael please get a cup of tea' is what he thought he heard. This may seem a slightly strange thing to happen; but how often in a clinical emergency have you asked for something and been presented with something else? People are less likely to ask questions in emergencies as everyone is busy. This could be the catalyst for an error or precipitate a missed task. So how do we find out what message Michael received? The easiest way is to include a feedback loop.

> Now the conversation goes:
> TEAM LEADER    'Michael, can you please connect the ECG?'
> MICHAEL          'Okay, just connecting the ECG'

We now know that the message has been transmitted and received correctly. For this process to work both parties (the sender and receiver) need to understand and expect it – again demonstrating the need for us to practise and train together.

## 4.7 Team working, leadership and followership

At a basic level a team is a group of individuals with a common cause. Historically we have tended to train individually or in professional silos, the risk here is that we are making a 'team of experts' rather than an 'expert team'. Often within healthcare our teams form at short notice and often arrive at different times. Much emphasis has previously been given to the role of the leader, but a leader cannot be a team on their own. As much emphasis should be given to developing the other team members, the active followers. A good leader will be able to swap from the role of leader to follower as more senior staff arrive and agree to take over.

### The leader

The leader's role is multifaceted and includes directing the team, assigning tasks and assessing performance, motivating and encouraging the team to work together, and planning and organising. All leadership skills and behaviours need to be developed and practised. There are different leadership styles and the leader needs to choose an appropriate style for each situation. Effective communication is key and should be reviewed and reflected upon regularly. Constructive feedback should both be given and sought in order to facilitate continuously improving performance.

### *Who is the leader?*

It is vitally important to have a clearly identified leader. There can be times when people come and go, or different specialties arrive, creating a situation where the leader may not be clear. In some situations or institutions, individuals will wear tabards or other forms of identification to mitigate against this uncertainty. If there is a scribe recording events they should record who is leading and any changes to the leader.

### *Physical position of the leader*

As soon as the leader becomes hands on and task focused, they are primarily concentrating on the task at hand. This becomes the focus of their thoughts and they lose situation awareness, their objective overview of the situation (see Section 4.7). The leader should be standing in an optimal position where they can gather all the information and ideally view the patient, the team members and the monitoring and diagnostic equipment. This enables them to recognise when a member is struggling with a task or procedure and to support them appropriately.

### Clear roles

Ideally the team should meet before the event and have the opportunity to introduce each other, and clarify roles and actions in emergencies. Sometimes this can be facilitated at the beginning of a shift but at other times it is impossible to predict or arrange. It is important, therefore, that individuals identify themselves to the leader as they arrive and roles are agreed, allocated and understood. A lot of the time their role maybe determined purely in relation to the specific bleep the individual carries, but it is important that team members are flexible, e.g. if three airway providers are first on scene we would expect other tasks also to be undertaken.

### Followership

The followers have roles that are as critical as the leader. Followers are expected to work within their scope of practice and take the initiative. No one would expect to turn up at a ward emergency and have a neat row of staff against the wall waiting for instructions. It is important to think about the level of communication required between the leader and followers. If it is obvious we are doing a task, this does not need to communicated. There is a risk that followers can overwhelm the leader with verbal communications where, in fact, the key is to communicate concerns or abnormal things. In the Formula One pit lane during a tyre change, the crew communicate (visually) as tasks are completed; they also signal if they have a problem, they do not communicate every expected step.

### Hierarchy

Within the team there needs to be a hierarchy. This is the power gradient; the leader is at the top of this as the person coordinating, directing and making the decisions. However, this should not be absolute. There is much discussion in the literature about the degree of the hierarchical gradient. If it is too steep, the leader has a massive position of power, their decisions are unquestionable and the followers blindly follow their orders. This is not safe because leaders are humans too and also make errors, their team is their safety net. Safe practice is achieved where the followers feel they can raise concerns or question instructions. This must always be understood by the leaders as much as by the followers. One way to reduce the hierarchy is for the leader to invite the team's thoughts and concerns, particularly around patient safety issues. It is also important for the followers to learn how to raise concerns appropriately.

One method that is sometimes used to raise concerns appropriately is **PACE** (probing, alerting, challenging or declaring an emergency). The probing question allows diplomacy and maintenance of the hierarchy whilst raising a point.

| Stage | | Level of concern |
|-------|---|------------------|
| **P** | Probe | *I think you need to know what is happening* |
| **A** | Alert | *I think something bad might happen* |
| **C** | Challenge | *I know something bad will happen* |
| **E** | Emergency | *I will not let it happen* |

These stages are described with examples below.

***Probe*** is used where a person notices something they think might be a problem. They verbalise the issue, often as a question: *'Have you noticed that this patient is cyanosed?'*

***Alert*** – the observer strengthens and directs their statement and suggests a course of action: *'Dr Brown, I am concerned, the patient is deeply cyanosed, should we start BVM ventilation?'*

***Challenge*** – the situation requires urgent attention. One of the key protagonists needs to be directly engaged. If possible the speaker places themselves into the eye line of the person they wish to communicate with: *'Dr Brown, you must listen to me now, this patient needs help with his ventilation'.*

***Emergency*** is used where all else has failed and/or the observer perceives a critical event is about to occur. Where possible a physical signal or physical barrier should be employed together with clear verbalisation: *'Dr Brown, you are overlooking this patient's respiratory state, please move out of the way I am going to ventilate him'.*

The PACE structure can be commenced at any appropriate level and escalated until a satisfactory response is gained. If an adverse event is imminent then it may be relevant to start at the 'Declaring emergency' stage, whereas a much lower level of concern may well start at a 'Probing' question.

Some industries have also additionally adopted organisation-wide critical phrases that convey the importance of the situation, e.g. 'I am concerned', 'I am uncomfortable' or 'I am scared'.

## 4.8 Situation awareness

A key element of good team working and leadership is to be fully aware of what is happening; this is termed situation awareness. It not only involves seeing what is happening but also captures how what is seen is interpreted and understood, and how decisions and plans are made.

Typically three levels of situation awareness are described:

Level 1 – What is going on?

Level 2 – So what?

Level 3 – Now what?

### Level 1

Consider level 1 – the basic level – we are prone to errors even at this level. Looking is an active process, the risk is seeing what is expected to be seen, rather than what is there. Figure 4.2 shows the similar package design of two different medications, making errors more likely.

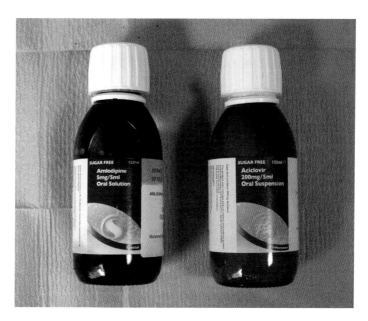

**Figure 4.2  Similar package design of two different medications**

It is important to really concentrate on seeing what is actually there.

### *Distraction*

Distractions in healthcare are so normal that individuals are often not even aware of them. The risk is that mistakes are made and information is missed. It is important to try to challenge interruptions when doing critical tasks and when they do occur restart the task from the beginning, rather than where it is considered the interruption occurred. Some organisations are looking at specific quiet areas for critical tasks. Whatever the local set up, the key is to develop and maintain everyone's awareness of how distraction greatly increases the chance of error.

## Level 2

Level 2 captures how the understanding forms of what has been seen. To minimise level 2 errors, consideration is needed as to how the human brain works and recognises things and how people make decisions and choices. This level of detail is beyond the scope of this introductory chapter, and therefore this section will focus on a part of this, the decision making that leads into level 3.

On the face of it the practice of decision making is familiar to everyone. However, to understand the factors that can compromise this process it is important to understand the factors that will influence the decision made. To make a good decision a person needs to assess all aspects of a problem, identify the possible responses to the problem, consider the consequences of each of those responses and then weigh up the advantages and disadvantages in order to draw a conclusion. Having completed this, they then need to communicate their decision to their team.

Good situation awareness is a basic prerequisite of this process. To achieve this, the decision maker must ensure they have all the key information. The whole team should be on the alert for ambiguities or conflicting information. Any inconsistent facts should be treated as a potential marker for faulty situation awareness. They should never be brushed off as unimportant anomalies in the absence of evidence to support such a decision.

In many clinical situations there can be a significant pressure of time. Where this is not the case, then no decision-making process should be concluded until the team is satisfied they have all the information and have considered all the options. Where time is limited, a certain amount of pragmatism must be employed. There is plenty of evidence to confirm that practise and experience can mitigate some of the negative effects of abbreviating a decision-making process. Individuals making decisions under such circumstances need to remain aware of the short-cuts they have taken. They should be ready to receive feedback from their team, particularly if any member of the team has significant concerns about the proposed course of action.

### Level 3

Having seen and understood, we can now plan forward and communicate this with the team.

The individuals in the team may have a different awareness of the situation depending on their previous experiences, specialty, physical position, etc. The team's situation awareness will often be greater than any individual's awareness, however this can only be exploited if the individual elements are effectively communicated. The leader should actively encourage this.

## 4.9  Improving team and individual performance

In addition to effective communication, team working, situation awareness and leadership and followership skills, there are a number of other ways that team and individual performances can be further developed and improved.

### Awareness of situations where errors are more likely

If we are aware that errors are more likely we can be more proactive in detecting them. Two common situations that make errors more likely are stress and fatigue. Stress is not only a source of error when we are overworked and overstimulated, but also at the other end of the spectrum when we are understimulated and become inattentive.

The acronym **HALT** has been used to describe situations when error is more likely.

| | |
|---|---|
| **H** | Hungry |
| **A** | Angry |
| **L** | Late |
| **T** | Tired |

**I'M SAFE** has been used as a checklist in the aviation industry asking whether the individual may be affected by the following:

| | |
|---|---|
| **I** | Illness |
| **M** | Medication |
| **S** | Stress |
| **A** | Alcohol |
| **F** | Fatigue |
| **E** | Eating |

Ideally, individuals who are potentially compromised need to be supported appropriately, allowed time to recover and the team made aware of the situation. How this can be achieved in the middle of a night shift though can be problematic.

### Awareness of error traps

A common trap that people fall into is only seeing or registering the information that fits in with their current mental model. This is known as a *confirmation bias*. When this occurs people favour information that confirms their preconceptions or hypotheses regardless of whether the information is true. This may be observed within the healthcare setting during the process of a referral or handover. An example of this might be a clinician receiving a phone call requesting them to attend the ward to review an acutely deteriorating patient. The clinician is advised that the patient is a known asthmatic. On their way to the ward the clinician builds up a series of preconceived expectations around what they will find upon their arrival. They may even formulate a management plan whilst travelling to the scene, based upon their expectations. Once this mindset is established it can be difficult to shift.

On arrival, the clinician examines the systems affected by the presumed diagnosis. They seek to confirm their expectation by focusing on an auscultation of the chest at the expense of a thorough assessment. Upon hearing bilateral wheeze their preconceived ideas are confirmed and the remainder of the assessment is completed without due attention and more as a rehearsed exercise rather than an open minded exploration. They fail to notice that the patient also has a soft stridor and is hypotensive. In this case the eventual diagnosis of anaphylaxis becomes at best a very late consideration, or at worst a situation that requires an objective newcomer to the team to point out the diagnosis.

**Cognitive aids: checklists, guidelines and protocols**

Cognitive aids such as guidelines are made available because the human memory is not infallible. They also confer team understanding through the use of a standardised response. This reduces stress. This is especially true where an uncommon emergency event occurs. The team may be unfamiliar with one another and each member will be trying to remember what to do, what treatments are required and in what order. A good team leader will use the available cognitive aids as a prompt and the team's members can use them as a resource so that they can plan ahead. Safe practice is promoted through the use of these tools in an emergency rather than relying on memory.

**Calling for help early**

Trainee staff are often reluctant to call for senior help, partly due to not recognising the severity of the situation but also due to concerns about wasting the time of seniors. With all emergency events, and in particular with paediatric emergencies, escalation and appropriate help should be summoned as soon as possible. Remember help will not arrive instantly.

**Using all available resources**

Team resources include staff, observations, equipment, cognitive aids and the facilities in the local area. The team leader should continually consider the appropriateness of utilising available, untasked staff or equipment to optimise the patient's care and prevent a bottleneck in the treatment pathway.

**Debriefing**

Wherever possible a debriefing should be facilitated, even briefly, following clinical events. Ideally this should be normal procedure, rather than being reserved for catastrophic events. The aim of a debrief is to summarise any particular issues or problems that the team had, and to reflect on how the team performed. Some organisations have set templates to facilitate this. It gives the opportunity for individuals, teams and organisations to continually develop.

## 4.10 Summary

In this chapter we have given a brief introduction to human factors that can lead to poor team working, patient harm and adverse events. It is really important for you to use every opportunity to reflect and develop your own performance and influence the development of others and the team. Appropriate debriefing is included in the scenarios for the NAPSTaR course which may be used to incorporate this process into your own clinical practice.

# PART 2
# The elements of transfer

| ACCEPT and SCRUMP principles | | | |
|---|---|---|---|
| **Assessment** | **S Shared assessment** | What is the problem? (think summary)<br>What is being done? (think background)<br>What is the effect? (think assessment)<br>What is needed now? (think recommendation) | |
| **Control** | | Identify team leader(s)<br>• Clinical<br>• Logistic<br>Identify and allocate tasks to be carried out<br>Pre-transport advice: ABCDEF | |
| **Communication** | | Communication – what:<br>• Who you are – contact details<br>• What the problem is (soundbite)<br>• Relevant details<br>• What you need from the listener<br>• What you have done<br>• Effect of these actions<br>• Summarise agreed plans<br>• What you need from the listener | Communication – with who:<br>• Local team<br>• Transfer team<br>• Receiving team<br>• Ambulance control<br>• Family |
| **Evaluation** | | Establish urgency of transfer<br>Is the transfer appropriate – going to the right place?<br>Speed and mode of transfer | |
| **Preparation Packaging** | **C Clinical isolation**<br>**R Resource limitation**<br>**U Unfamiliar equipment**<br>**M Movement and safety**<br>**P Physical/physiological changes)** | Checks of patient, equipment and personnel | |
| **Transportation** | | Handover – CLEAR | |

# CHAPTER 5
# Assessment

---

**Learning outcomes**

After reading this chapter, you will be able to:
- Describe a systematic approach to gathering key information and undertake an assessment of the clinical needs of the patient
- Understand the logistics required for transfer

---

## 5.1 Introduction

The clinician leading a potential patient transfer may have had no contact with that particular patient before being called by the treating clinical team. It is vital for the person taking responsibility for coordinating the transfer to learn how to assess such a situation quickly and effectively. This must be done before becoming directly involved with the patient's clinical management, and it may include providing advice to the referring team regarding ongoing resuscitation and stabilisation.

A proper assessment requires knowledge of the patient's condition and of the actions of the treating team, the results of those actions and the capabilities of the transferring team. The answers to several key questions will help this process (Box 5.1).

---

**Box 5.1  Assessment questions**

- What is the problem? (think summary)
- What is being done? (think background)
- What is the effect? (think assessment)
- What is needed now? (think recommendation)

---

## 5.2 Formulating the assessment

A careful enquiry should be made into the history of the current illness or injury, i.e. 'What are the problems?' Many clinicians will be familiar with SBAR (situation, background, assessment and recommendation – see Chapter 7). The 'What are the problems?' question could be considered to be equivalent to the situation part of SBAR.

Ideally, a referral form (see Appendix D) should be used to ensure that all the key information is gathered. Where this is not available, an ABCDEF approach should be adopted to identify the immediate and predicted clinical needs of the patient.

The question 'What is being done?' (which could be considered as being equivalent to background in SBAR) provides the opportunity to check that appropriate treatment, if not already being undertaken, has been started.

The effect of any intervention should be evaluated ('What is the effect?'). This question could be considered to be equivalent to the assessment part of SBAR.

---

*Neonatal, Adult and Paediatric Safe Transfer and Retrieval: A Practical Approach to Transfers*, First Edition.
Edited by Bernard Foëx, Peter-Marc Fortune and Cassie Lawn.
© 2019 John Wiley & Sons Ltd. Published 2019 by John Wiley & Sons Ltd.

All of the information from these enquiries should provide the basis of how to answer the next question: 'What is needed now?' (which could be considered as being equivalent to recommendation in SBAR).

Throughout the process continuous re-evaluation of the status of the patient, in particular the effect of clinical interventions, should be undertaken. Ask the question 'Is what is being done, working?' If not, what is needed to improve the patient's clinical status? It will usually be possible to stabilise the patient for transfer. Following this, the role of the transfer team is to further optimise the conditions, and forward plan in order to achieve a safe transfer to the ward, unit or department for ongoing care.

Handover and communication of clinical information will be required at least once and often multiple times during the transfer process. This should be undertaken in a structured way using a focused 'soundbite' that succinctly describes the situation.

## 5.3 Summary

Assessment is the essential first step to identify problems and actions required to plan ongoing care.

# CHAPTER 6
# Control

## 6.1 Introduction

It is important that a clear structure of command and control is both present and understood within every transport team.

## 6.2 Controlling the situation

Following the initial assessment, someone needs to take control and coordinate ongoing activity. This involves:

- Identifying the clinical and logistical team leader
- Identifying the tasks to be carried out
- Allocating tasks to individuals or teams

### Identifying the clinical and logistical team leader

A clinical and logistical team leader (or multiple leaders) needs to be identified. If there is one individual as leader, they will be the overall lead for the transfer. If there are two or more individuals, one of them needs to be identified as overall lead. The clinical lead takes responsibility for ensuring that the patient's clinical care is appropriately delivered. The logistical lead has responsibility to deal with the communications, resources and logistics of the transfer.

If there are two different individuals taking the clinical and logistical team lead roles, then one of these individuals must be identified as overall transport lead. Clear communication between the clinical and logistical leads is essential.

As well as being present, the transfer team leader/s must have sufficient experience to be capable of successfully seeing the task through and must be experienced enough to have the confidence of other members of the team. In any given situation, an appropriate leader or leaders is usually obvious, because of either a person's experience, seniority or both. If this is not the case, the most experienced member of staff present should take this role initially, whilst seeking senior or more experienced help.

### Identifying the tasks to be carried out

Whilst control is established, clinical care of the patient must continue without interruption, and communication with other key personnel becomes a priority. The resources that must be secured, including staffing, equipment and necessary drugs will need to be identified and brought to the patient. This process can be summarised in a general task list. This list is a generic starting point and should be expanded and developed for individual clinical situations (Box 6.1).

*Neonatal, Adult and Paediatric Safe Transfer and Retrieval: A Practical Approach to Transfers*, First Edition.
Edited by Bernard Foëx, Peter-Marc Fortune and Cassie Lawn.
© 2019 John Wiley & Sons Ltd. Published 2019 by John Wiley & Sons Ltd.

**Box 6.1  General task list**

- Continue direct patient care
- Communications
- Collect the equipment and resources that will be needed

**Allocating tasks to individuals or teams**

Tasks should be delegated by the transfer team leader to appropriate personnel. Competence is the key attribute and tasks should only be given to staff that have the appropriate training and expertise. The team leader/s will need to consider the relative priority of each task and the scope for concurrent activity.

## 6.3  Summary

Whilst many teams function in a fluid manner, passing responsibilities from one person to another, it is crucial that a recognised command structure is present to unambiguously coordinate team activity.

# CHAPTER 7
# Communication

---

### Learning outcomes

After reading this chapter, you will be able to:

- Recognise who should undertake communication and who they should communicate with
- Define what needs to be communicated
- Describe some of the communication methods used in transfers
- Identify the methods of ensuring successful communication

---

## 7.1 Introduction

As has already been stated, the successful transfer of an ill or injured patient from one clinical area to another requires the coordinated effort of many individuals from a number of different teams. Good communication is essential to achieve the cooperation and coordination of these people.

Good communication is:

- Structured
- Complete
- Concise
- Clear and unambiguous

It should be:

- Friendly and respectful
- Open minded

It should employ:

- Feedback and confirmation

The communication process begins as soon as the initial referral begins. The clinician receiving the call must facilitate effective communication with those who are already dealing with the patient so that an accurate picture is drawn up. It is this picture upon which the initial assessment will be carried out. Good communication between professionals must continue through the control phase to the point when the decision to transfer is made. At this point the need for transfer must be communicated to all other teams who need to be consulted or who will become directly involved with the patient's care. The appropriate receiving clinical area should be identified as soon as possible. In many cases the transport will need to be organised after the receiving team has formally agreed to accept the patient. However, centralised specialist transport teams will often mobilise their team immediately after referral; the process of identifying and securing the receiving bed is then undertaken concurrently with the team's mobilisation.

Given the requirements detailed above, communication is placed at the heart of the ACCEPT approach. Throughout the transfer good communication remains an essential part of the process. Both the referring and receiving teams must be kept informed, as must the transport providers. Relatives and supporting services must also be kept up to date at all stages of the

---

*Neonatal, Adult and Paediatric Safe Transfer and Retrieval: A Practical Approach to Transfers*, First Edition.
Edited by Bernard Foëx, Peter-Marc Fortune and Cassie Lawn.
© 2019 John Wiley & Sons Ltd. Published 2019 by John Wiley & Sons Ltd.

transfer. This is particularly important where the patient is a child. It is good practice to advise the patient's relatives when and how they can expect to hear updates on progress (text, phone, face to face). The relatives should be provided with a single point of contact during transport. Ideally, this should be either at the referring or receiving centres rather than the transport team who may be distracted from key tasks by calls en route. Throughout the entire process an accurate record of activity and communications should be maintained in either a written or electronic form.

Many different methods of communication may be employed during the transfer. Initially (at the referring unit), most of the communication will be face-to-face or by telephone. Once the transport is underway mobile phones and radios may be used. Finally, face-to-face communication with the receiving team will be important, as will the delivery of an accurate written or electronic record. Texts and instant messaging systems may be a useful adjunct to other forms of communications but these media are particularly prone to misinterpretation and must be used with great care.

The clinician responsible for the decision to transfer the patient holds the ultimate responsibility to ensure all appropriate communication takes place. Similarly, the accepting clinician in the receiving unit has ultimate responsibility for ensuring that the handover communication at that end of the transfer chain is both unambiguous and sufficient. These clinicians may have to delegate some of the calls to other members of staff. Key calls, such as those offering and accepting the patient, should be made between those with clearly identified responsibilities for the question at hand. Even if calls are delegated, it is important that the outcome is reported to the responsible clinicians at each unit so that they maintain an overview of the transfer process.

## 7.2 What needs to be communicated?

Successful communication has only occurred when *all* the necessary information has been passed on and understood by *all* the relevant people. During the transfer process, successful communication requires that both clinical and transportation arrangements are made and understood. As already noted, each communication episode should consist of the following:

- Who you are
- What the problem is
- What the (relevant) patient details are
- What you need from the listener
- What you have done to address the problem
- Effect of these actions
- Summarise agreed plan
- What is needed from the listener

The above components may be captured in an SBAR structure if staff are familiar with using this tool. Further details on this tool may be found at: https://improvement.nhs.uk/resources/sbar-communication-tool/ (accessed December 2018).

### Who you are (contact details)

Not only should the instigators of the call identify who they are, they should also state whether they are calling on their own behalf or if they have been assigned the task of communication by someone else. This ensures that the receiver of the call has a clear idea as to whether the call has been instigated at an appropriate level, helping to avoid misunderstandings later on. Sometimes the most senior clinician will be actively involved with the patient's clinical care and may need to delegate the call to a more junior team member.

### What the problem is (soundbite)

This is closely related to the patient's needs, and the details required will vary. For example, communications designed to book an intensive care bed will be very different from those to an ambulance service to arrange elective transportation. In the first instance considerable clinical information may be required, and the exact amount will be a matter of negotiation between the instigator and the receiver of the call; in the second, much less information is needed. This negotiation is an important aspect of the call; as a starter, the instigator should prepare a concise verbal presentation of the clinical details.

Much time is wasted during telephone referrals when every request for additional information is followed by a need for further communication with a third party in the background. The need for this can be reduced by the availability of summary notes written in the style of a form that captures the key information, as discussed in Chapter 5.

## What the (relevant) patient details are

The exact details that are relevant will vary with the nature of the need. However, a minimum dataset consists of:

- Patient's full name
- Patient's date of birth or age
- Patient's current location

Many receiving units have a proforma to collect the necessary information. If these are also made available to referring units it allows them to collect all relevant information in the format in which it will be required. A national or regional form is ideal, where available.

## What you need from the listener

This is the most important part of the call from the perspective of both the caller and the listener. It is therefore essential that the need is stated clearly and succinctly. For example: *'My patient needs an intensive care bed'*.

## What have you done to address the problem and effect of these actions

If the communication is designed to obtain clinical services, then the treatment given, and the response to that treatment, will be very important in completing the picture for the receiver of the call. They need to assure themselves that all appropriate measures either have been undertaken, or are in the process of being undertaken. For example:

- What has been done? – use an ABCDEF approach
- What was the effect of these interventions? – use an ABCDEF approach

This is especially important when the referral is to a specialist service, since the early delivery of good care will help to ensure that the patient arrives in the best possible condition.

In paediatric and neonatal practice it is an integral part of the role of the specialist transport service to provide advice to the referring unit throughout the transfer process.

## Summarise agreed plan and what is needed from the listener

Summarise the agreed plan. Since the statement of need is so important, it is recommended that it is restated at the end of the communication so that no misunderstandings occur, e.g. *'So, I need an intensive care bed'*.

## 7.3 Communication with who?

The following should be communicated with:

- Local team
- Transfer team
- Receiving team
- Ambulance control
- Family

The clinician responsible for the patient's care is ultimately responsible for all communications about the medical management of their patient. Some key communications around the request for and acceptance into specialist care, including intensive care, must be made directly at a senior level. Other communications may be delegated to one or a number of members of the team. However, the team leader has a responsibility to ensure that all those who need to be communicated with are contacted and that messages are timely, clear, concise and consistent. If more than one person is involved in communication, it is important that a structured approach, as outlined in this chapter, is used in order to avoid confusion. It is also important to inform the team leader and record the outcome of all communications. A list of some of the calls that may be necessary during the transfer process is given in Table 7.1 together with a list suggesting which staff could be asked to make them.

**Table 7.1** Calls made during transfer

| | Nature | Responsibility |
|---|---|---|
| Transfer calls | Seek availability of bed | Clinician or administrator |
| | Book transport | Clinician or administrator |
| | Communicate with receiving department or unit | Clinician or administrator |
| | Arrange staff: | |
| | Nursing | Nurse |
| | Ambulance | Clinician or administrator |
| | Medical | Doctor/transport practitioner |
| Clinical calls | Discuss with specialist | Doctor/transport practitioner |
| | Negotiate bed | Clinician |
| Information calls | Inform responsible consultants | Doctor/transport practitioner |
| | Inform relatives | Clinician |

## 7.4 Communication methods

The communication methods used during the transfer process are the same as those used during day-to-day practice. The usual method within the clinical area instigating the transfer is face-to-face speech, while most other communications (within both the referring hospital and the receiving unit) are by telephone.

### Written (electronic) records

Written records are especially important from both the clinical and legal perspectives. Apart from a few taped calls, written notes are usually the only records that remain once the transfer is completed. They must be both as accurate and contemporaneous as possible and should include as a minimum:

- Patient demographics
- Timings
- Clinical baseline history and examination
- Clinical interventions and effects of these interventions
- Investigations carried out and their results
- Condition during transfer
- Names of responsible clinicians at each stage of the transfer

In addition, a written record of the actual transfer process should be completed. All entries must be signed, dated and timed. Where handwritten entries are made the clinician's name should be clearly printed under their signature together with their role and professional registration number.

### Handing over

Handover and communication of clinical information will be required at least twice and often many more times during the transfer process. All such communications should start with a summary of the problem. In many cases this will be easy to capture succinctly; however, where patients have a complex medical history that is more difficult to summarise, it is essential that the focus is on key information pertinent to their current clinical problems. Additional background information should also be available for discussion but not necessarily volunteered in the initial summary. All of the information must be documented in a logical, presentable and reproducible format that is made available to all of the clinicians that assume responsibility for the patient's care.

During the transfer process itself, the patient's active problem will need to be communicated to a number of people in a short space of time. Acute clinicians are often working under pressure and are distracted by, or intolerant of, long-winded explanations. The use of an attention grabbing 'soundbite' is a useful technique to capture the salient features of a complicated story into a short sentence of fewer than 15 words. It should be an easily repeatable description that captures the most relevant aspects of the case. Mastering the soundbite takes practise. It is worth silently rehearsing with all the patients you see. Following the soundbite introduction, a succinct ABCDEF description of what has been done, and its effect, should precede the request for transfer.

### Feedback loop and summarising – what you need from the listener

It is good practice to make use of feedback and microsummaries throughout all communications to ensure that the person you are talking to has interpreted the key information in the way you intended.

A microsummary can be interspersed in conversation, by the speaker (person transmitting the information), to re-emphasise key points. For example at the end of a discussion of required therapy the speaker might say *'So, we have agreed to administer 10 ml/kg of normal saline, start gentamicin and secure a review from your local cardiologist'.*

Feedback is not dissimilar to a microsummary in content but originates from the listener (the person receiving information) and thus effectively confirms that both parties are on the same page.

### Ambiguities and confusing information

It is not uncommon for some aspect of a communication to embrace more than one possible action or simply not to make sense to the receiver. It is well known that sometimes people can be reluctant to revisit such information at the risk of looking stupid. Often the receiver assumes that all will become clear later. This is never a safe position and it is particularly risky during a transfer process where there may be no way to clarify the information, or nobody present to help untangle understanding should it be required. Therefore, ALWAYS ensure that you understand all that is said to you and challenge any information that is unclear or ambiguous.

## 7.5 Summary

Clear and effective communication and documentation are essential parts of the transfer process. All key parties must be kept up to date at all times and any gaps in understanding or ambiguities should be addressed immediately.

# CHAPTER 8
# Evaluation

### Learning outcomes

After reading this chapter, you will be able to:
- Recognise and agree to the need for transfer
- Evaluate the transfer category

## 8.1 Introduction

Evaluation is a dynamic process that starts from the first contact with the patient. The aims are to decide whether transfer is appropriate and, if it is, the priority of the patient in comparison with other clinical demands. By the time assessment, control and communication have been completed, enough information will have been gathered to make such an evaluation.

## 8.2 Recognising and agreeing the need for transfer

The possibility of transfer on clinical grounds requires recognition that the needs of the patient may have to be met elsewhere. In order to make this decision the likely, or possible, diagnoses must be identified and the indicated investigation or treatment for such conditions must be known. The lack of local facilities, resources or personnel to make the definitive diagnosis and/or to treat the condition optimally must be recognised and suitable acceptable alternatives need to be available. Referral patterns and common indications for clinical transfers will be well known in most units. In many cases the transfers will be undertaken for expertise or facilities that are best managed by regional or supra-regional specialist services. However, some referrals will be made because of a lack of capacity in the referring unit or for repatriation to a hospital nearer to a patient's home.

Having identified the possible need for inter-hospital transfer, the duty clinician at the regional specialist transport service or receiving centre should be contacted. Local practice will dictate which of these are appropriate. A two-way dialogue will usually result in an agreement that transfer is appropriate. Sometimes immediate agreement is not possible and further information is required: for example, a neurosurgeon may need to assess a computed tomography (CT) scan transmitted electronically from the referring centre. Occasionally, agreement to transfer is not achieved because of a very poor prognosis (e.g. 80% burns in an elderly patient) or it is deferred until stabilisation has been achieved to permit safe transfer. On these occasions the regional transport services will usually be able to continue to provide advice and support to the referring centre. Sometimes teams are mobilised to support the referring team.

After agreeing about the appropriateness of transfer, the retrieval/receiving clinician must check that the receiving centre is able to accept the patient. Necessary resources (such as intensive care beds) should be confirmed as being available. This rule may be over-ridden when the receiving centre has the capability to perform an emergency life-saving surgical (now also radiological) intervention which is critically time dependent. In such a situation, transfer prior to availability of resources may be justified but the specialist receiving centre will have to arrange further transfer postoperatively. A good example of this would be a neurosurgical intervention for an expanding intracranial lesion.

*Neonatal, Adult and Paediatric Safe Transfer and Retrieval: A Practical Approach to Transfers*, First Edition.
Edited by Bernard Foëx, Peter-Marc Fortune and Cassie Lawn.
© 2019 John Wiley & Sons Ltd. Published 2019 by John Wiley & Sons Ltd.

## 8.3 Transfer category

This is the next stage in the process and represents part of the dialogue between the referring, transferring and receiving clinicians. The need for extra treatment prior to or during transfer should be discussed and an assessment of the urgency of transfer made. A primary goal of safe transfer is to move the appropriate treatment environment with the patient. Thus, for transfer of an intensive care patient, the ambulance should function as a mobile intensive care unit.

A useful tool for determining the appropriate transfer needs is the transfer category table (Table 8.1). The patient's illness or injury is identified in such a way as to incorporate severity and urgency. It provides a consistent method of allocating resources (vehicle, escorts and equipment) and defining the ambulance response time.

**Table 8.1** Clinical urgency

| Category of clinical incident | Urgency | Vehicle | Driving speeds | Personnel |
|---|---|---|---|---|
| Major trauma | As 'Emergency – unstable' and in compliance with local major trauma network guidelines | | | |
| Emergency | Unstable | TIME CRITICAL Mobilise team in less than 30 minutes Local team may need to be mobilised sooner | Transport team ambulance or '999' ambulance Consider air transfer if this significantly reduces journey time without engendering significant delay | Use of blue lights and sirens to maintain normal progress advised Driving with exceptions may be indicated | Competent neonatal/ adult/paediatric transport clinician and nurse Often local team to avoid delay |
| Emergency | Stable | Mobilise team in less than 30 minutes | Transport team ambulance or '999' ambulance Consider air transfer if this significantly reduces journey time without engendering significant delay | Use of blue lights and sirens to maintain normal progress advised Driving with exceptions may occasionally be indicated | Competent neonatal/ adult/paediatric transport clinician and nurse Occasionally local team to avoid delay |
| Urgent | Ill and stable | Mobilise team in less than 60 minutes | Transport team or '999' ambulance | Normal road speeds. Use of blue lights and sirens to maintain normal progress may occasionally be indicated | Clinician competent in age appropriate BLS. Usually this will be a nurse, but may be just the paramedic crew |
| Elective | | Arranged 1–2 days in advance | Transport team ambulance or other appropriate ambulance, e.g. patient transport service vehicle or '999' ambulance | Normal road speeds | Transport nurse and/ or transport clinician depending on clinical situation |

## Box 8.1  Categories of clinical urgency

- Major trauma
- Emergency – unstable (*Time critical*) (**Time critical**)
- Emergency – stable (*Intensive*) (**Uplift of care**)
- Urgent (ill and stable) (**Capacity transfer**)
- Elective (planned) (**Repatriation**)

The clinical urgency is divided into five categories (Box 8.1). The terminology used differs slightly between adult and paediatric/neonatal practice. Where this is the case the paediatric terms are shown in *italics* and the neonatal categories are shown in **bold**.

## Major trauma

Major trauma patients will not always present or be brought directly to a major trauma centre (MTC). They will need a secondary transfer to an appropriate MTC. Depending on their injuries they may need a time critical transfer, in which case they will require a similar response from the ambulance service as a 999 (or European 112) call. An example is a patient with a traumatic brain injury who has needed intubation because of airway compromise. Such patients will need to be escorted by a doctor and a nurse who are both competent in transfer medicine. Some patients may be considered as emergency stable, for example those with a spinal injury and no respiratory or cardiovascular compromise.

## Emergency – unstable (time critical)

Time critical transfers involve patients requiring the most urgent transportation. These transfers require a similar response time from the ambulance service as a 999 (or European 112) call. An example is a patient with evidence of a ruptured abdominal aortic aneurysm or with a traumatic brain injury, with no access to facilities to perform surgery on site. Delaying to attempt stabilisation is of little or no benefit. Transferring such patients requires an advanced life support provider, who may be a paramedic, a specialist nurse or a doctor. All paediatric and neonatal transfers will require a doctor or advanced transport practitioner on the team. However, this is not always the case for adult transfers where a paramedic may fulfill the same role.

## Emergency – stable (intensive)

Although intensive patients are usually the most complicated (often requiring ventilation and invasive monitoring), they are not necessarily the most urgent. Careful stabilisation prior to transfer is important.

For those working outside a service with dedicated transport, a proactive decision should be made to request an ambulance to be made available at an appropriate time. At the very least, in a relatively simple case, it will takes 20–30 minutes to establish the patient on a transport ventilator and repeat blood gas analysis to confirm appropriate settings. In an ideal world an ambulance should be ordered in time to avoid unnecessary delay once the team is ready. However, the ambulance service is also heavily stretched and it should not be ordered so far in advance that the vehicle and team have to wait too long. This ideal can be difficult to achieve!

An example of such an intensive case is a child with severe meningococcal septicaemia requiring transfer to a paediatric intensive care unit. Resuscitation fluids, inotropes and antibiotics will have been given already, arterial and central venous lines inserted and intubation performed. Intensive patients will often require advanced respiratory support and advanced monitoring techniques. Frequently, more than one organ system will need support. The transfer team should include a doctor and a nurse trained in critical care. Ideally both should also be familiar with the transport environment.

## Urgent (ill and stable)

Transfer within 60 minutes is desirable but may be flexible in order to respond to other, more urgent calls on specialist staff and transportation.

Ill and stable patients constitute the majority of medical and surgical patients admitted to hospital for acute care on a daily basis. Examples include patients with a chest infection without serious respiratory compromise; a stroke without airway obstruction, irregular breathing or hypotension; or acute appendicitis without perforation. Neonatal patients such as those with suspected necrotising enterocolitis may also fall into this category.

This category of patient may be considered stable enough not to require the presence of an advanced life support provider en route if transferred. Nevertheless, transport staff must always be competent in basic life support skills appropriate to the age of the patient. Adults and children in this group are ill and will require a stretcher rather than a seat in an ambulance. A BabyPod™ or incubator should be used for newborns and small infants. Ill patients will usually be accompanied by a nurse in addition to the ambulance team. Some adults may be transferred by a paramedic crew only. A decision to transfer without a nurse escort should always be in line with local policy and sanctioned by the supervising medical team.

### Elective (planned)

Adult patients classified as unwell or well are included in the table for completeness but will not be discussed further here. They form an important part of the overall transport requirements within a large hospital (especially intra-hospital rather than inter-hospital transfer) but require fewer special arrangements.

Stable neonates may also fall into this category when being transferred for reviews, treatment such as cryotherapy for retinopathy of prematurity, and repatriations. These patients can represent a significant proportion of neonatal transfers and will usually be accompanied by a neonatal nurse at all times.

## 8.4  Summary

Evaluation of the patient is a continuous process that starts from the first medical contact. It aims to determine the rationale for and the urgency of transfer.

# CHAPTER 9
# Preparation and packaging

---

**Learning outcomes**

After reading this chapter, you will be able to:
- Describe how to prepare the patient, equipment and personnel for transfer
- Explain the importance of a structured approach to the preparation and packaging of a patient for transfer

---

## 9.1 Introduction

Following initial assessment and rectifying any potentially life-threatening problems, reassessment and planning of definitive care will need to be undertaken; this will include ensuring that the patient is prepared for transportation. Even moving a patient from the emergency department to a ward requires planning for the patient's current needs and the potential needs en route.

The acronym **MINT** may be used to remind the team that 'preparation and packaging' does not only involve the physical preparation and continued treatment of the patient, but involves the preparation as well as the packaging of the medical and nursing staff who may accompany the patient. Instrumentation refers to the need to bring together all the equipment required to monitor and treat the patient during transportation. Transportation is a reminder of whether the patient is to travel by cot, bed, incubator, hospital trolley or ambulance trolley. Thought must be given in advance to the practicalities of being able to observe and access the patient and their attendant equipment and ensuring that the whole package is safe both for the patient and the accompanying staff.

---

**MINT**

**M**   Medical
**I**    Instrumentation
**N**   Nursing
**T**    Transportation

---

## 9.2 Preparation

There are three distinct areas that require preparation before packaging can be commenced:

- Patient – The patient must be stabilised to reduce physiological complications during the journey
- Equipment – All the necessary equipment must be found, be appropriate for transport use and be checked
- Personnel – The personnel who are to undertake the transfer must be fully prepared

---

*Neonatal, Adult and Paediatric Safe Transfer and Retrieval: A Practical Approach to Transfers*, First Edition.
Edited by Bernard Foëx, Peter-Marc Fortune and Cassie Lawn.
© 2019 John Wiley & Sons Ltd. Published 2019 by John Wiley & Sons Ltd.

## 9.3 Patient preparation

Before the transfer, the team leader must ensure that the patient is physiologically optimised and that all team members are fully briefed about the patient's needs. Optimisation of the patient's condition will normally be synonymous with physiological stability. However, there will be occasions when the need for transfer to a specialist centre requires the transport team to continue stabilising manoeuvres en route. An example of this might be a hypoxic child, with a severe pneumonia or pneumonitis, on high ventilator pressures and 100% oxygen being transferred to a paediatric intensive care unit for high frequency oscillation.

Once again the ABCDEF approach is used. The patient must have a 'definitive' airway. If there is any doubt whatsoever about the patient's airway or level of consciousness, then elective intubation should be considered and undertaken prior to departure. As a guide, anyone with a Glasgow Coma Scale (GCS) of 8 or less should usually be intubated prior to transfer, unless there is a good reason not to do so. Most children requiring transfer will be intubated and any decision not to intubate a child should only be taken in concert with the supervising consultant. The need to intubate en route should not arise. If it occurs, it should be the subject of a detailed debrief and/or incident investigation as dictated by local policy.

The cervical spine should be immobilised in patients with a known unstable neck injury; this may involve head blocks (Figure 9.1), sand bags or a vacuum mattress, and where possible axial loading must be avoided. Spinal boards should only be used in the short term for extrication: scoop stretchers should be used to assist with transportation and transfer (Figure 9.2).

Even in patients without cervical injury, it is still often worth stabilising the head during transfer. A vacuum mattress is particularly useful in this regard, particularly when transporting children.

To stop the head rolling, bags of fluid or rolled towels may be placed on either side of the head but they do not offer effective cervical spine protection.

> **Head blocks, sand bags or a vacuum mattress offer the best immobilisation of an unstable cervical spine during transportation**

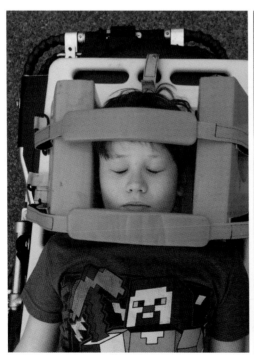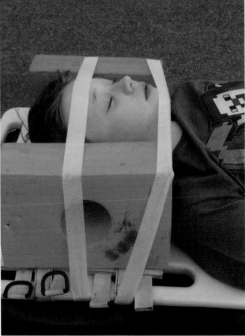

**Figure 9.1  Head blocks and tape.** Courtesy of Mark Woolcock

(a)

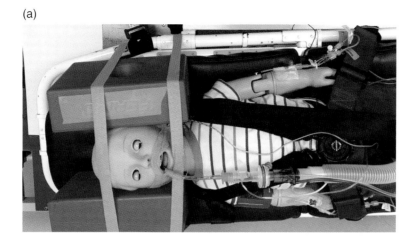

(b)

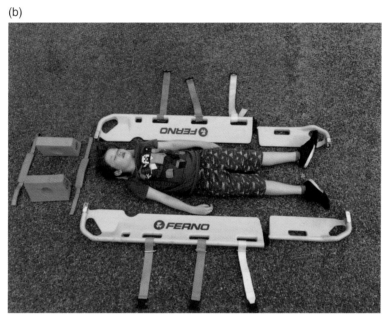

**Figure 9.2 (a) Child on a scoop stretcher.** Courtesy of Kate Parkins. **(b) Scoop stretcher.** Courtesy of Mark Woolcock

Spontaneously breathing patients that require supplementary oxygen should continue to receive this. It is essential that these patients are monitored using pulse oximetry (at the least). Appropriate calculations should be undertaken to ensure sufficient supplies of gas are available to achieve this for twice the anticipated length of time (see Chapter 18). Suitable masks or nasal speculae, including a non-rebreathing mask, should always be available in case the patient deteriorates. Sometimes adult patients requiring high concentrations of inspired oxygen are much better transferred sitting up, with an appropriate securing harness.

Chest drains can present an additional challenge if the transfer includes an ambulance journey. Underwater seal bottles are cumbersome, can tip over or spill and should not be used on the road. One-way valve drainage bags provide a suitable alternative although a compromise solution may be required if the volume of drainage is significant.

Ideally, at least two reliable sites of intravenous access should be available. In children a secure multilumen central line may be considered sufficient. In any case where it is difficult to secure a second line of access an EZ-IO™ drill and needle may be considered as a back up (Figure 9.3). (An interosseous needle may even be used as primary access where an alternative solution cannot be sited within an appropriate time frame.)

Maintenance fluids should be administered to most patients. However, for patients over 2 years of age they may be omitted for shorter transfers. Most fluids should be administered via a suitable infusion pump or syringe driver: these will be far more effective than a free-flowing drip set whilst in motion. Transfers may take longer than expected, and maintenance fluids should always be available even if not initiated at the beginning of the journey. Infusions should be rationalised in order to

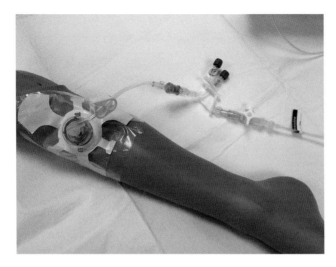

**Figure 9.3 EZ-IO™ needle in situ with proprietary dressing.** Courtesy of Kathryn Claydon-Smith

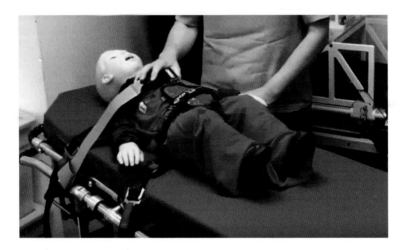

**Figure 9.4 Patient secured to stretcher with a harness.** Courtesy of Kathryn Claydon-Smith

reduce the number to a minimum. When many infusions are required or intravenous access is at a premium it may be possible to give as a bolus rather than infuse some agents such as muscle relaxants or sedatives. Essential infusions, such as inotropes or vasopressors, should continue to be administered by continuous infusion.

The patient has to be appropriately packaged for transport. In all cases patients must be suitably secured to the trolley or bed, using an appropriate device or harness (CEN (European Committee for Standardisation) compliant) (Figure 9.4). All fractures must be immobilised prior to transport.

Any suspicion of a spinal injury, at any level, warrants appropriate spinal immobilisation during transport. Spinal boards offer excellent immobilisation; however, there is a high incidence of pressure sores with prolonged spinal board use. Placing a full length, pressure relieving gel pad, of the type used in the operating theatre, may help to protect the skin, whilst maintaining immobility. Vacuum mattresses are a useful alternative to spinal boards (Figure 9.5): they must be secured to the trolley and patient immobility confirmed prior to departure. It is important to note that some pelvic fixators and traction devices may not fit into the transport vehicle and may require modification or removal.

Patients of all ages, especially small children and babies, may become hypothermic whilst being resuscitated and stabilised for transfer. Efforts should be made to minimise exposure during invasive procedures in order to reduce heat loss. Warm air quilts and other methods should be used to maintain an appropriate temperature throughout stabilisation and transfer. For neonates and small babies, this may be facilitated using an incubator or pod. Chemical gel mattresses may be employed for infants and small children during the transfer. See Chapter 14 for further details on warming.

(a)                                    (b)

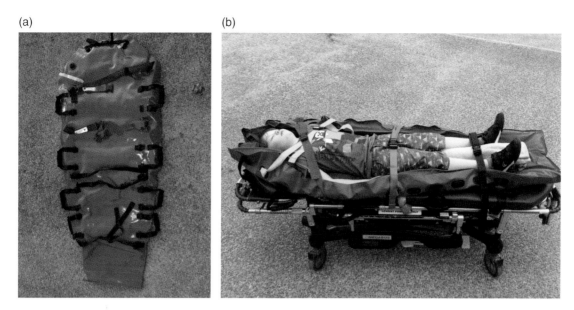

**Figure 9.5 (a) Vacuum mattress. (b) Vacuum mattress in use.** Courtesy of Mark Woolcock

## 9.4 Equipment preparation

### Patient equipment

Transport equipment should be kept separate from other supplies to ensure it is always immediately available for use. It should be stored in a specific location and must be checked regularly. Monitors and pumps must be kept fully charged in accordance with manufacturers' instructions to maximise battery life. Some items require storage in different conditions and therefore may be held in different locations, for example drugs that are stored cold, warmed fluids, controlled drugs and batteries on charge. These can easily be forgotten and it is therefore important to use a pre-departure checklist.

Most hospitals will have transport bags or trolleys that are specially designed to ensure that staff can quickly find the equipment they require. It is important that they are designed so that they can be secured in an ambulance whilst still providing rapid access to the equipment they contain. A number of these systems use smaller pouch bags with specific uses such as 'airway' or 'intravenous access' (Figure 9.6). When moving critically ill patients over long distances, a great deal of equipment may be required. Spreading the load between two smaller transport packs may be better than using one large one, depending on local arrangements. The requirements of air transfers present different challenges of weight, space and access. Ideally, the kit would be identical for both air and land transfers, however this is not essential. The key is familiarity with the equipment being used.

After each transfer, the transport kit must be restocked and repacked against a checklist. Keeping a record of any items used during a transfer can streamline this process, but is not a substitute for the checklist process. Many teams choose to seal bag compartments after restocking to indicate to everyone that they contain a complete set of equipment.

The kit must contain all means of manually supporting the airway, and full intubation equipment for all appropriate ages and conditions. This should include a selection of sizes of masks, airways and endotracheal tubes. The inclusion of advanced airway kit should be considered. Effective portable suction must be available at all times. Hand or foot operated units can be very efficient for large volume suction and have the advantage of needing no external power or gas supply. Oxygen supplies and devices are dealt with in detail in Chapter 18.

A mechanical ventilator should be used for all patients requiring ventilatory support. This must be durable, safe and reliable. Many of the suitable portable ventilators are gas driven and therefore it is important to consult the tables provided with the machine to ascertain their total gas consumption. All intensive care patients require a ventilator that can cope with a variety of lung conditions. A ventilator that can provide positive end expiratory pressure (PEEP) is essential for all children's transfers.

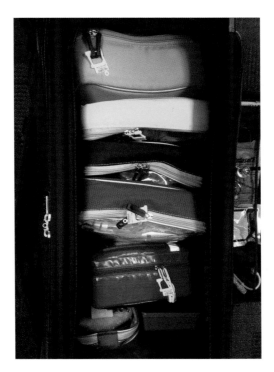

**Figure 9.6 Transport bag containing role-specific pouch bags.** Courtesy of Kathryn Claydon-Smith

It is important to ascertain the total oxygen requirement for the transport episode. This can be calculated as follows from the following information:

- Flow rate of oxygen (to mask, or total consumption of ventilator) (litres/min)
- Total journey time; comprising of sum of times (minutes) for:
  - Moving from ward to ambulance
  - Loading ambulance
  - Travel
  - Unloading ambulance
  - Moving from ambulance to ward.

If part of the journey is in another vehicle (e.g. aircraft) a further load time, travel time and unload time will need to be accounted for. This amount should then be **doubled** to allow for unforeseen problems.

Consider the following example of a ventilated patient:

- Requirement: 100% oxygen
- Tidal volume ($V_t$) of 0.8 litres
- Rate of 13 breaths per minute

The patient's minute volume is easily calculated as tidal volume multiplied by rate ($0.8 \times 13$), i.e. 10.4 l/min. Consulting the ventilator manual shows that the device itself consumes 1 l/min of gas to drive the system. So the total oxygen consumption will be 11.4 l/min.

The team plans to use an E-sized oxygen cylinder (680 L) to transport the patient to the ambulance, a journey which may take up to 20 minutes. Inside the ambulance, they plan to use one of the two F-sized cylinders (1360 L each) for the 50 minute journey. On arrival at the receiving hospital the team will revert to the E-sized cylinder and has planned to allow 25 minutes for this leg of the journey. This information is summarised in Table 9.1.

The team should check that the ambulance does have at least one full F-sized cylinder, which should be sufficient for the 45 minute journey, with an adequate reserve. However, the single E-sized cylinder leaves little margin for error, especially if the gas consumption has to be increased by using a bag and valve circuit if the ventilator malfunctions.

**Table 9.1** Oxygen consumption calculation

| | Time in minutes | O₂ consumption (l) based on 12.2 l/min | O₂ consumption (l) based on 15 l/min |
|---|---|---|---|
| a) To the ambulance | 15 min | 183 | 225 |
| b) Loading ambulance | 5 min | 61 | 75 |
| c) In the ambulance | 50 min | 610 | 750 |
| d) Unloading ambulance | 5 min | 61 | 75 |
| e) From the ambulance | 20 min | 244 | 300 |
| Total while mobile on trolley (a + b + d + e) | 45 min | 549 | 675 |
| Total while inside ambulance (c only) | 50 min | 610 | 750 |
| Grand total | 95 min | 1159 | 1425 |

In the worst case scenario, unexpected delays may occur en route, or an unnoticed leak or a failure to close the flow valve after use may completely exhaust a cylinder of any size. Therefore it is good practice to always carry at least twice the anticipated amount of oxygen required split between at least two cylinders (Table 9.2 and Figure 9.7).

In the event of a ventilator failure it must be possible to attach a breathing circuit to an alternative gas port; this will require either a second cylinder with the appropriate connections, or a combination regulator that has provision for Shräder *and* nipple outlets. In addition, a self-inflating bag should always be available in case of failure of both of the ventilator and gas supply.

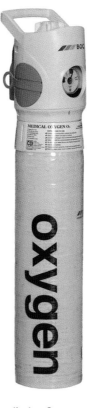

**Figure 9.7 Oxygen cylinder.** Courtesy of BOC Healthcare

**Table 9.2** Capacity of different size cylinders

| Cylinder size | Capacity (litres O₂) |
|---|---|
| C | 170 |
| D | 340 |
| CD (lightweight) | 480 |
| E | 680 |
| F | 1360 |

Under exceptional circumstances, the ambulance may have to stop en route at a hospital or ambulance station to collect more oxygen. This should always be avoided if it is possible to safely carry enough oxygen for the entire journey. Either way, a reserve is essential for unexpected delays or when transporting from isolated locations, where additional supplies cannot be collected during the journey. Teams should consider including a regular cylinder check along with their patient observations to ensure gas supplies do not unexpectedly run out. For long transfers and premature babies it is important to consider the risks of administering oxygen at excessive levels. Some transport ventilators cannot entrain enough air to reduce the inspired oxygen content toward that of air. Where lower concentrations are required, a suitable ventilator must be used; this will normally require a compressed air supply. Some specialist vehicles will have compressors on board to deliver this supply. However, if this is not available then appropriate calculations must also be made for air supplies and sufficient cylinders of air carried to deliver this requirement.

Some highly specialised transfers may require further equipment checks, e.g. incubators, extracorporeal membrane oxygenation machines and portable balloon pumps. These may necessitate an appropriate technician joining the team. The additional team member must be fully briefed on the patient, the transfer and details of the transport environment, e.g. power and gas supplies on board.

### Staff equipment

All transport team members must wear a protective, high visibility jacket suitable for work outside the safety of the hospital. The team should have the ability to communicate by telephone and carry appropriate resources to ensure that they can make their own way back to the base if necessary. A simple mnemonic checklist is shown in Box 9.1.

---

**Box 9.1 PERSONAL equipment**

| | |
|---|---|
| **P** | Phone and charger |
| **E** | Enquiry number and name |
| **R** | Revenue |
| **S** | Safe clothing |
| **O** | Organised route |
| **N** | Nutrition |
| **A** | A–Z (map/SatNav) |
| **L** | Lift home |

---

## 9.5 Personnel preparation

Staff who are tired, hungry and travel sick are unlikely to provide optimal care during transfer. Motion sickness can be a genuine problem for transport staff, not only because of discomfort to the staff, but because of proven poor performance in these circumstances. Those who suffer from motion sickness should try simple measures – such as travelling forwards, travel sweets, looking at the horizon, avoiding looking at screens, sitting in front (when possible) and keeping well hydrated – to try to alleviate the problem when they are not the primary carer for a patient. Antiemetics can also be helpful and some staff find elasticated acupressure travel bands beneficial.

Staff involved in any transportation of patients must have the skills and competencies appropriate to deliver the level of care required by the patient, and be familiar with the idiosyncrasies of the mode of transportation. The clinical needs of a stable patient being transferred within the hospital are usually met by a qualified ward nurse. However, an intensive inter-hospital transfer will require advanced skills and a team of two or three. A guide to the competencies required for transfer medicine can be found in the standard document published by the Paediatric Intensive Care Society Acute Transport Group and the *Guidelines for the Transport of the Critically Ill Adult* published by the Intensive Care Society. Good communication between transport staff is critical in achieving a safe and efficient transfer.

## 9.6 Packaging the patient

The key goal in packaging the patient is to achieve both physical security and accessibility. Equipment must be secured to the patient; the patient secured onto the stretcher, pod or incubator and, in the case of ambulance transfers, the stretcher, pod or incubator secured into the vehicle (Figure 9.8). Staff should think ahead when packaging the patient, and bear in mind where they will be located in relation to the patient. Access to the patient is often compromised in some way once in the back

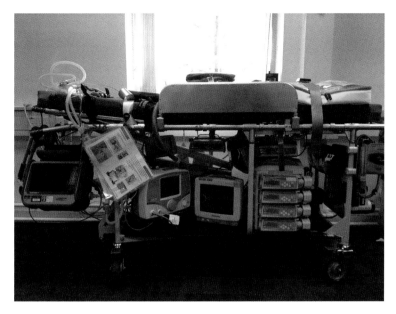

**Figure 9.8 Specialised transport trolley with all key equipment attached.** Courtesy of Kathryn Claydon-Smith

of a vehicle. In most cases, the team will sit either at the head end or on the patient's right side. In most ambulance configurations access to the patient's left side is difficult if not impossible. Physical and visible access to airway, breathing and circulation devices and equipment should be considered during packaging. The addition of extension sets to left-sided intravenous lines should be used to provide access to the patient's circulation if suitable lines are not available on the right.

Similarly, patients undergoing magnetic resonance imaging (MRI) or computed tomography (CT) scans will need to be observed from a remote control room. In these cases intravenous access is frequently required for the administration of radio-opaque contrast; this carries the risk of anaphylaxis which, although remote, should be planned for.

Having formulated plans for access during transportation, equipment must be secured to the patient. The use of the systematic ABCDEF approach to securing and checking should be used. All endotracheal (ET) tubes must be securely fastened. In adults this usually means using a cord tie or cotton tape, but care must be taken to avoid neck compression, especially in head-injured patients. Children's ET tubes should be secured with Melbourne strapping and neonatal tubes according to local policy (usually using a proprietary device). Ideally, all small children should have a nasal rather than an oral tube. This is easy to secure and less prone to loosening from tapes becoming wet with secretions. In adults, ET tubes should be cut to the correct length. In children and neonates the additional length may permit more flexibility when packing the patient. In any case excessively long tubes may kink, especially if they are of a small diameter and attached to a heavy ventilator circuit. Splitting a larger tube and using it to strengthen the length protruding from the mouth or nose can add some rigidity and therefore resilience in this regard.

## Melbourne strapping technique

In order to prevent skin damage caused by adhesive tape, the child's skin should be protected with a proprietary skin protecting adhesive dressing such as DuoDERM®. Such dressings consist of a flexible, polyurethane, outer foam layer and an adhesive skin contact layer which contains a moisture absorbing hydrocolloid material.

The taping procedure is classically described for nasal intubation and comprises the use of three separate pieces of adhesive tape. The application procedure is described here.

1. Cut a length of string slightly longer than the distance around the child's face from one ear to the other
2. Tie the string around the ET tube with a single knot positioned posteriorly (Figure 9.9). The tube may then be held securely in place by an assistant holding the string
3. Prepare the skin protecting patches: to affix directly to facial skin use DuoDERM® or equivalent
4. Use strips of Sleek® or Elastoplast® to prepare two 'trouser legs' and one 'eyehole'. The trouser legs need to be long enough to pass across the nose and wrap around the ET tube. Each trouser leg must have a thick and a thin limb (Figure 9.10)
5. Place the DuoDERM® patches on the face on either side of the nose to protect the skin (Figure 9.11)

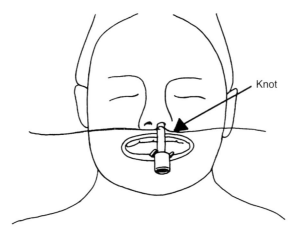

**Figure 9.9 Tie the string around the tube**

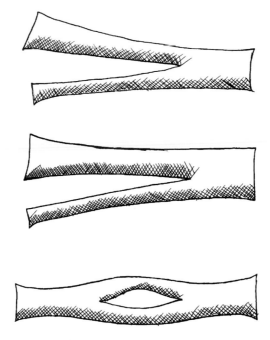

**Figure 9.10 Adhesive tape preparation: two trouser legs**

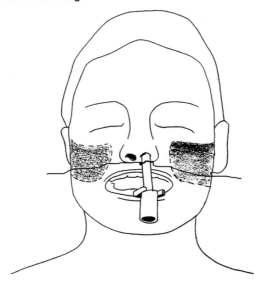

**Figure 9.11 Application of DuoDERM® skin protection**

6. Place the wide part of the first trouser leg, over the stretched string, on the side of the face furthest from the ET tube. Apply the inferior trouser leg under the nose and onto the DuoDERM® patch on the other side (Figure 9.12a)
7. Stretch and apply superior trouser leg over nose and around the ET tube. The tape should pass from nose to tube at lateral edge of nares as shown (Figure 9.12b).

(a)                                                       (b)

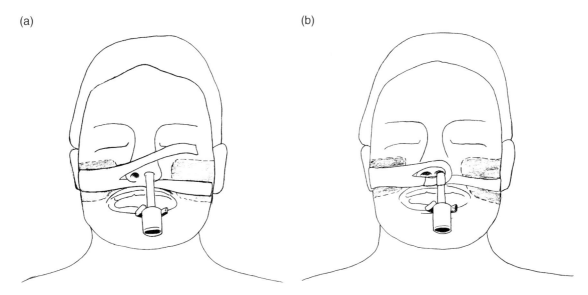

**Figure 9.12  Application of first trouser leg: (a) inferior leg under the nose, and (b) superior leg wrapped around the endotracheal tube**

8. Repeat the same procedure starting with the wide part of the second trouser leg passing from the same side as the ET tube. On this occasion the superior leg passes over the nose and onto the opposite cheek (Figure 9.13a)
9. The inferior leg is stretched up, and around the ET tube, from below (Figure 9.13b)

(a)                                                       (b)

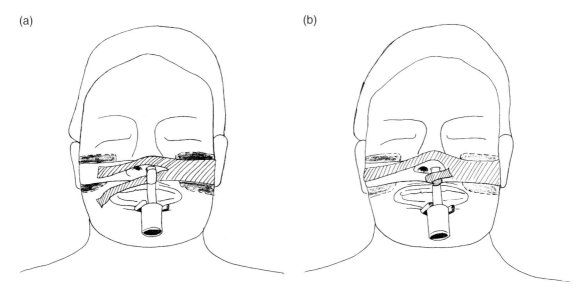

**Figure 9.13  Application of second trouser leg: (a) superior leg over the nose, and (b) inferior leg wrapped around the endotracheal tube**

10. Place the 'window tape' over the previous tapes, ensuring that the maximum visibility of skin surface around both nostrils is achieved. Note that the application is most easily achieved by removing the ET tube connector to prevent catching
11. Finally, replace the ET tube connector (Figure 9.14)
12. On completion, the majority of the circumference of the intubated nostril should remain visible for inspection

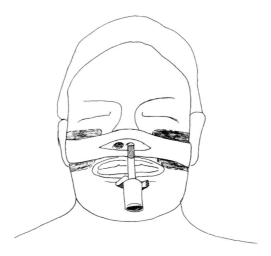

**Figure 9.14 Replacement of the endotracheal tube connector**

The ET tube must be controlled and monitored at all times with the goal of preventing unintended extubation. The risk of this is highest when moving the patient between platforms such as the bed and transport trolley or onto the MRI table. If the patient will tolerate a short period off the ventilator, then it is recommended that the ET tube is disconnected from the ventilator circuit during such manoeuvres in order to minimise the risk of snagging the circuit and causing an unintended extubation.

If the atmospheric pressure is likely to change significantly, for example during air transport, the cuff on the tube (if present) should be filled with saline rather than air. This will avoid the associated volume changes that can damage the trachea and/or burst the cuff. Good practice should always include a regular check of the cuff inflation pressure in order to detect any issues early.

## 9.7 Packaging equipment

Ventilators and associated equipment need to be thoroughly checked and tested prior to departure. The entire transport team must be familiar with the ventilator being used and all of its alarms. The ventilator circuit should be secured to prevent dragging on the catheter mount and ET tubing. The ventilator and any oxygen cylinders should be fastened securely to the stretcher or transport trolley. They should ideally remain clearly visible and be easy to reach at all times. Ventilator pressure and disconnect alarms can be very difficult to hear during transport. If fitted, they should be used, but they should not be relied on. Extra vigilance to tube issues is essential throughout the transfer. For this the gold standard is continuous end-tidal $CO_2$ monitoring. This must be employed for all intubated patients (see later in this chapter).

The content gauge of the oxygen supply must be clearly visible and monitored regularly. A reserve oxygen supply must be readily available and should have an appropriate connector attached. When using cylinders that require a key to turn them on, the key becomes an essential part of the kit that should be included on the check list and it needs to be readily available.

Adequacy of respiratory support is assessed by capnography and pulse oximetry. The oximeter probe can be attached to a suitable site inside the patient's blankets or wrap, to reduce the effect of ambient light. Clip-on probes that are taped onto a finger or toe can lead to pressure necrosis and should be avoided. Self-adhesive probes are very useful, especially in the paediatric and neonatal population, and function well in vibrating environments. Ear probes are rarely of value for transport purposes. Capnography is an essential component of respiratory monitoring and should be closely monitored. Care should be taken to ensure that if an in-line sensor is used, its weight is supported in order to reduce drag on the ET tube.

### Lines

When securing lines prior to transfer, remember that when the patient is covered or wrapped, one point of venous access should be kept easily available to avoid delays in giving drugs. Jugular and subclavian central lines often provide good points of access for a carer sitting near the head of the patient. Femoral or umbilical lines are often used in children and care must be taken to ensure ready access to these lines is maintained once the patient is fully packaged. For neck lines the access port can be secured to the pillow or shoulder of the patient to avoid displacement during the journey. It is good practice to clearly identify the contents of an intravenous line by labelling at the patient end.

## Monitors

Many sensors may be required to monitor the patient's physiological status. This results in a potentially huge jumble of cables and wires. To avoid this all the leads should be brought together as one bundle, held together with some short lengths of split plastic tubing or tubular bandage. The whole bundle can be threaded out of the coverings, pod or incubator to the monitor(s).

Invasive pressure sets should be bubble free and checked to ensure that all connections are appropriately tightened. Do not over tighten connections as this can result in damage or difficulty releasing them when required. Transducers should be flushed and zeroed prior to use. If equipment is moved around or the readings do not make sense, they should be re-zeroed at the earliest safe opportunity. Pressure transducers can be fastened to the chest (children) or right upper arm (adults), which will be nearest to the transfer team members in the ambulance, where they are readily accessible for flushing and zeroing. Transducers must also be secured at an appropriate level for monitoring cardiac pressure. Gauze may be placed under each transducer before taping to the patient, or proprietary fixing solutions used, to prevent pressure necrosis.

It may be possible, with prior discussion, to arrange for power for monitors and pumps to be drawn from the ambulance. Some of these devices may be able to operate at 12 V, e.g. transport incubators. If this is not the case an inverter is required, which converts 12 V DC to 240 V AC. Ad hoc use of an inverter is not recommended as it is relatively easy to compromise electrical safety if it is not installed by an appropriately qualified engineer. Many ambulances have an inverter fitted as standard and AC is available.

In terms of packaging for disability, the eyes of sedated patients must be protected with tape, gauze or gelatin patches. This should prevent accidental corneal abrasion but should be applied in such a way as to allow visualisation of the pupils, both for neurological observations and to assess sedation levels.

Heat loss outside the warm hospital environment can present a major problem, especially in children. For neonates and small infants this can be partially mitigated by the use of a pod or incubator. Older children or adults should be adequately covered and may be 'mummy wrapped' by completely surrounding them with a blanket. This technique is rarely used in children because the requirement to secure them to the trolley with a five point harness precludes this approach. Pre-warmed blankets may be used and covered with an insulating layer where available. Alternatively, quilts or sleeping bags can be used for maximal insulation. The thermal environment inside the transport vehicle should also be considered. It should be possible to arrange for the ambulance to be pre-heated before loading the patient. This is absolutely essential for neonates and small children who will become hypothermic in a cold ambulance even if they are themselves within a pod or incubator.

Many teams will choose to move the patient onto the transport trolley at the beginning of the packaging process and then 'pack around them'. This is essential when an incubator is used that is likely to be permanently attached to the transport trolley. The stretcher and the secured and covered patient must then be secured in the ambulance (Figure 9.15). The whole stretcher system and ambulance must be CEN compliant: able to withstand decelerations of up to 10 G, without the stretcher moving significantly.

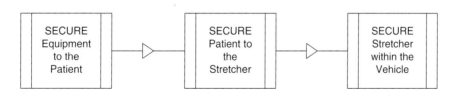

**Figure 9.15 The stages of securing**

Safely securing the equipment to the stretcher or trolley usually requires some form of commercially available, CEN compliant, mounting. This is to ensure that in the event of a rapid deceleration, medical equipment such as monitors or syringe drivers do not become high velocity lethal missiles.

The current most popular design consists of a fixed height stretcher with secure mountings for the monitor, oxygen cylinder, ventilator and syringe drivers which are located within the rigid trolley chassis underneath the patient mattress.

## 9.8 Summary

Adequate preparation of the patient, the equipment and the transport personnel, together with attention to the details of packaging, will ensure that the transportation phase itself has the best chance of being free of adverse events.

# CHAPTER 10
# Transportation

---

## Learning outcomes

After reading this chapter, you will be able to:
- Describe the final actions necessary before leaving the referring unit
- Identify potential problems that may require action during the transfer
- Identify the actions necessary on arrival at the receiving unit

---

## 10.1 Introduction

Inter-hospital transportation takes place in three distinct phases. Firstly, the patient is moved from the referring unit to the transferring vehicle. Secondly, the vehicle, team and patient move from the referring unit to the receiving unit. Finally, the patient is moved from the transferring vehicle to the receiving unit trolley or bed. These three phases are dealt with separately below.

## 10.2 Leaving the referring unit

The patient and transfer team should be fully prepared and packaging must be complete before any movement is initiated. A final check should be carried out to ensure that no final actions are required to ensure stabilisation. In addition, a final check should be made to ensure that tubes, drains and lines are as secure as possible. Box 10.1 shows the sequence of actions that should occur. A checklist should be used at this stage to optimise compliance.

---

### Box 10.1 Checklist prior to leaving the referring unit

The patient may be moved into the incubator or onto the trolley at the beginning or end of this sequence according to the team's normal practice

1. When transporting a neonate ensure the incubator is pre-warmed before moving the baby into it
2. If the patient is not intubated, change to a transport oxygen supply and ensure the incubator, high flow humidified nasal specs or mask is set up and fits appropriately
3. Ensure the transport oxygen cylinder is full and has the appropriate valve(s)
4. If requiring ventilation, attach the patient to the transport ventilator to check adequate ventilation and oxygenation are achieved; check blood gases before departure
5. Ensure adequate ventilation to both sides of the chest
6. Ensure any chest drain is secure and functioning and appropriately terminated
7. Check that any bandages providing tamponade are secure
8. Ensure intravenous lines are secure, untangled and functioning
9. Hang up any fluid bags so they will not interfere with the transfer of the patient
10. Check the position of the urinary catheter and position it between the patient's legs or on the trolley as appropriate
11. Check the position of the naso/orogastric tube and position the bag on the patient appropriately
12. Plan the move with the team and ensure all key parties are briefed
13. Warn the patient (if appropriate)
14. Check that no line, tube or cable is likely to be snared in the move
15. Notify receiving unit of estimated time of arrival

---

*Neonatal, Adult and Paediatric Safe Transfer and Retrieval: A Practical Approach to Transfers*, First Edition.
Edited by Bernard Foëx, Peter-Marc Fortune and Cassie Lawn.
© 2019 John Wiley & Sons Ltd. Published 2019 by John Wiley & Sons Ltd.

## 10.3 Movement between units

The aim is to provide seamless, appropriate care throughout the transfer. Using a systematic ABCDEF approach will identify potential problems that may require action during the transfer. There are many potential problems during any transfer, some are specific to the clinical condition of the individual patient, the equipment being used or the mode of transport.

For each of the systems (physiological, technological and logistic) undertake a pre-transfer check before leaving. Consider what the potential threats are, how the risk of these occurring can be minimised and what would be the warning signs of imminent or actual occurrence. For each issue identified agree a plan of action in order to prime the team to respond coherently, promptly and efficiently.

---

**Identify threats and agree actions**

**What could go wrong?**

**Plan a systematic (ABCDEF) approach to:**

- **Identify incipient/actual problems promptly**
- **Prevent events cascading into a major event (if possible)**
- **Take pre-planned action should a major issue occur**

---

## 10.4 Airway

Before setting off perform a pre-transfer check of the airway system (Box 10.2).

---

**Box 10.2 Pre-transfer checklist – airway**

Will it be possible to assess the airway during transfer?

Is there a member of the team present who can secure that airway, if required?

*If the patient is intubated*:

- Is the ET tube visible?
- Is the ET tube adequately secured?
- Is the length of the tube at the lips or nose recorded?
- Is the pilot balloon visible and pressure checked (if present)?
- Are the connections to the ventilation tubing visible and secure?
- Does a member of the team have access to the drugs and equipment that might be needed?

---

The most serious threat to the airway is a total loss of control because of disease progression (in an unintubated patient with upper airway pathology) or displacement of an endotracheal (ET) tube. The patient with an unsecured airway may also rapidly deteriorate or vomit and aspirate gastric contents or blood and ET tubes may migrate inwards or become blocked with secretions.

### Simple monitoring

In the spontaneously breathing patient, observing the ease of breathing and looking for the signs of obstruction can be extremely difficult in a moving ambulance; this is even more difficult if the patient is mummy-wrapped or transported in an incubator or pod. Listening for sounds of obstructed breathing or ET leaks in a ventilated patient is also difficult because of the amount of noise within an ambulance or a fixed wing aircraft, and is impossible in a helicopter. However, despite the problems, simple physical monitoring techniques should not be abandoned as, when possible, they are often far more resilient than technological solutions.

### Pulse oximetry and capnography

Pulse oximetry gives a continuous measurement of the level of tissue oxygenation at the probe site. The first sign of an airway problem during transfer may be a deterioration in the oxygen saturation. That said, pulse oximetry measurements can be unreliable during transfer. For example, if the patient is cold and peripherally vasoconstricted, the signal strength may not be sufficient to give an accurate reading of oxygen saturation. Furthermore, readings can be distorted by vibration artefact and excessive ambient light.

The ability to measure arterial $CO_2$ is not available to most teams during transfer. Proprietary bedside blood gas analysers are available but are generally only carried by specialist teams. However, end-tidal $CO_2$ measurement using capnography is widely available and will give a constant indication of the adequacy of ventilation in the intubated patient. The capnograph can also act as an extremely sensitive disconnection alarm since the trace will disappear almost immediately once the patient is no longer ventilated. This is important since the alarm systems of transport ventilators can be variable in their response times. Capnography should be considered a basic standard for all intubated patient transfers.

In-line capnographs can be affected by moisture build-up within the sampling window; side stream capnographs may also cease to work if the sampling tube becomes blocked with moisture. Both pulse oximetry and capnography are described in more detail in Chapter 18.

## Threats to the airway

### *Outward migration of the endotracheal tube – dislodgement*

Despite the best efforts to secure it adequately, the ET tube may become dislodged. Outward dislodgement of the ET tube will usually exhibit the signs of a leak. An early sign may be a gurgling sound on inspiration; if so, check that the level of the tube at the lips or nose has not changed from the recorded value. As the tube migrates out there may be a loss of the gurgling sound, but also loss of ventilation. Check the ventilator's pressure dial and the end-tidal $CO_2$ trace.

---

**Actions**

- Stop the moving vehicle as soon as possible and assess the patient
- If possible, confirm displacement by direct visualisation; if in doubt remove the ET tube
- Ventilate via bag–valve–mask technique
- Reposition the ET tube or reintubate as indicated
- If close to the end of the journey, there is no risk of aspiration and it is easy to ventilate by mask consider completing the journey with bag-valve-mask support

**NB** Notify the receiving centre and lead consultant of the situation as soon as possible

---

### *Inward migration of the endotracheal tube – endobronchial intubation*

Inward migration of the ET tube may mimic the signs of a tube obstruction. The first indication may be a high inflation pressure seen on the ventilator dial or a fall in oxygen saturations as a result of ventilating only one lung. Check the ventilation pressure dial and the pulse oximeter reading and check that the level of the tube at the lips has not changed from the recorded value. Be aware that if the ET tube appears to be secured at the correct level, and has not migrated, a pneumothorax should be ruled out.

---

**Actions**

- Stop the moving vehicle as soon as possible and assess the patient
- If possible, confirm displacement by direct visualisation (clear movement at the lips or nose to a longer length is sufficient confirmation in children and babies)
- With all the appropriate equipment available, reposition the ET tube and secure the tube

---

### *Endotracheal tube cuff leak (where used)*

The leaking of an inflated ET tube cuff may be detected by listening for a gurgling sound on inspiration, a loss of pressure on the ventilator or reduced chest movement. Any of these signs may alert the team to the problem, but other causes should also be considered. Undetected, a significant loss of inspired minute volume will result in hypoventilation, and eventual hypoxia and hypercarbia. The pulse oximeter should give a relatively prompt indication provided that the patient is not receiving an excessive amount of inspired oxygen. The end-tidal $CO_2$ trace will usually change but may not indicate hypercarbia; this measurement is unreliable with a large leak and may show a normal or even a low end-tidal $CO_2$ even when $PaCO_2$ has risen. It is vital to recognise that the space around a deflated cuff allows the aspiration of secretions, blood or gastric contents to contaminate the bronchial tree.

---

**Actions**

- Stop the moving vehicle as soon as possible and assess the patient
- Check that the level of the tube at the lips has not changed from the recorded value
- Attempt to introduce more air/saline into the cuff
- If the pilot balloon is damaged, introduce more air/saline into the cuff and clamp the pilot tube with artery forceps
- If the pilot balloon is lost consider introducing a 22 G cannula into the pilot tube and reinflating the balloon
- Consider replacing the ET tube completely

---

### Endotracheal tube obstruction/occlusion

Endotracheal tube 'blockage' as a result of inward migration has been discussed. Small diameter ET tubes, despite being well secured, can kink especially when the ventilator circuit is allowed to drag. Obstruction can also occur as a result of secretions drying within the ET tube which may be exacerbated when dry oxygen is used to ventilate the patient. Obstruction may be indicated by an increase in inflation pressure on the ventilator dial when there is an obstruction or kinking of the tube. A failure to overcome this obstruction can result in inadequate ventilation of the patient's lungs, especially when dealing with the small diameter tubes needed for paediatric patients. Use of a humidifier or heat moisture exchanger will reduce this complication.

---

**Actions**

- Stop the moving vehicle as soon as possible and assess the patient
- Visually check the ET tube for kinks
- Use the suction device and an appropriate suction catheter to clear secretions from the ET tube lumen
- Consider stopping the ambulance and replacing the ET tube completely

---

## 10.5 Breathing

Before setting off perform a pre-transfer check of the breathing system (Box 10.3).

---

**Box 10.3 Pre-transfer checklist – breathing**

If the patient is ventilated:
- Is the patient settled on and compliant with the ventilator?
- Do you have visual and hands-on access to the ventilator and the breathing circuit?
- Can you see symmetrical chest movement?
- Can you see the pulse oximeter and capnograph displays?
- Is a manual breathing circuit easily available?

---

As outlined in the Section 10.4, simple monitoring by looking and listening may be difficult to undertake in a moving vehicle. Most transport ventilators display airway pressure on an aneroid dial or digital display. Not all transport ventilators have low and high pressure alarms, although these should now be regarded as mandatory. A low pressure alarm is helpful in suggesting an airway disconnection or leak. High pressure alarms, when set correctly, may warn of a tension pneumothorax or airway obstruction (from tube kinking, bronchospasm or secretions).

### Threats to breathing

#### Pneumothorax

The potential for developing a pneumothorax is higher in certain patients. Children with chronic lung disease and/or reactive airways chest disease or older children/adults with asthma or chronic obstructive pulmonary disease (COPD) are likely to have bronchospasm. Immunocompromised patients with pneumocystic chest infections are at risk of barotrauma and pneumothorax. Patients with a history of trauma, which may have involved the chest, and those who have had attempted or successful central venous cannulation of the jugular or subclavian veins are at risk. It is important to note that the presence of a pre-existing chest drain can give a false sense of security, since a pleural leak can occur at another site, or the existing chest drain can become obstructed. Also, a chest radiograph performed after the insertion of the central venous line cannot exclude the possibility of a pneumothorax developing during transfer. The use of high inspiratory ventilator pressures will increase the risk of a pneumothorax in any patient. Adequate sedation and the use of muscle relaxants can ensure ventilator compliance and avoid coughing which increases intrathoracic pressure and risk of pneumothorax. There is no contraindication to the use of muscle relaxants during the transfer of an intubated patient.

Pneumothorax can be life threatening in a ventilated patient but is difficult to confirm in a moving ambulance or aircraft. Noise levels can make any attempt to assess air entry into the lungs by auscultation with a stethoscope futile. Transillumination of the chest may be possible in a neonate or small child. It is important to ensure that any light source used for this is suitable and will not burn the child. Tracheal shift is an unreliable, very late sign which may be impossible to assess in a neonate or small child. A rise in the inflation pressure on the ventilator dial may be the only sign that a pneumothorax has developed. Hypoxia, as demonstrated by a pulse oximeter, may occur only shortly before an elevated central venous pressure, and a catastrophic fall in blood pressure may be seen on the monitor as a tension pneumothorax develops. If you suspect a pneumothorax is developing stop the ambulance, look and percuss for hyper-resonance and transilluminate as appropriate (Box 10.4). The treatment of a pneumothorax is discussed in some detail in *Advanced Paediatric Life Support* (APLS), 6th edition (Samuels and Wieteska, 2016).

---

### Box 10.4  Pneumothorax detection in the transfer of a ventilated patient

- Have a high index of suspicion in at-risk patients
- React early to any rise in ventilator inflation pressure
- Exclude a blocked or kinked ET tube
- Check any existing chest drain is not kinked
- Stop the ambulance and undertake a thorough check for hyper-resonance and/or transilluminate the child's chest

---

As an emergency measure, a 16 G cannula (smaller in an infant or child) connected to a 10 ml syringe may be inserted into the second intercostal space in the mid-clavicular line on the suspected side, or the side demonstrating most hyper-resonance. It may be impossible to reach the fourth intercostal space in the mid-axillary line on the patient's left side, and in the 'mummy-wrapped' patient it is difficult to use this approach on the right. Some centres recommend the use of a Veress™ laparoscopic insufflation needle. The aim is to decompress the chest (a more detailed description is available in the APLS 6th edition manual). Inserting a conventional chest drain during an ambulance journey is fraught with problems; in such circumstances consideration should be given to the use of a Seldinger guidewire chest drainage system. The guidewire may be passed directly through an ordinary cannula; however, note that the guidewire will not pass through a Veress needle.

---

**Actions**

- Stop the ambulance
- Confirm signs
- Insert a cannula into the second intercostal space mid-clavicular line and aspirate air
- Recheck the ventilator and monitors
- If successful consider converting to a chest drain

---

### *Lung ventilation and perfusion mismatch*

This occurs during transfer because the blood flow in the relatively low pressure system of the lung is influenced by acceleration and deceleration forces. This may result in the patient becoming hypoxic. Extra oxygen must be added to compensate for the increasing intrapulmonary shunting of deoxygenated blood. Oxygen should be titrated throughout the transport to ensure appropriate oxygenation (usual $SpO_2$ of 94–98%, but lower in some children with cyanotic congenital heart disease). Small variations may be attributed to this phenomenon; however larger swings should prompt a systematic search for the underlying cause.

### Loss of oxygen supply

Loss of oxygen supply not only reduces the $FiO_2$ but may also stop the transport ventilator working altogether, since many transport ventilators are gas powered. Prevention is much better than cure and although some causes, such as faulty seals, are unpredictable, the commonest cause is failure to take enough oxygen (Box 10.5) (see Chapter 18).

---

#### Box 10.5 Prevention of loss of oxygen supply

- Calculate the amount of oxygen for each part of the journey before departing
- Check that the required supplies are available
- Ensure that at least two oxygen cylinders are carried
- Know where the cylinder key is stored and/ or how to turn the cylinder on
- Keep spare Bodok seals in your transfer equipment
- **Have an appropriate sized self-inflating bag available at all times**

---

## 10.6 Circulation and organ perfusion

Powerful inertial forces are well known to affect the cardiovascular system in healthy subjects. Hypovolaemic patients are more sensitive and may adversely respond to the inertial forces experienced transiently during an ambulance transfer, due to rapid venous pooling of blood in the peripheral tissues. Although little research exists, it is known that volume loading of the hypovolaemic patient reduces the incidence of tachycardia and reduced cardiac output. It is therefore important to ensure that the patient is adequately fluid resuscitated and that any potential source of blood loss is controlled. However, the team should bear in mind that in certain circumstances overaggressive fluid resuscitation may actually increase blood loss. During stabilisation resuscitation, the transfer team will have to balance the concepts of permissive hypotensive resuscitation against the adverse effects of inertia on the hypovolaemic patient.

It is important for the transfer team to have access to a range of monitoring parameters in order to evaluate the effects of the transfer environment on organ perfusion and the cardiovascular system (Box 10.6).

---

#### Box 10.6 Pre-transfer checklist – circulation

- Can you assess the patient's circulatory status?
- Do you have adequate IV access?
- Can you respond to changes in the patient's circulatory status?

---

The electrocardiogram should be monitored routinely during critical care transfer. At least three electrodes are required, allowing two for sensing and one as a ground. Some monitors use more electrodes to allow flexible switching between leads. The electrodes should be placed appropriately to facilitate interpretation. Positioning them in adults to provide the equivalent of standard leads II and V5 is useful for detecting P-waves/arrhythmias and myocardial ischaemia, respectively.

Invasive *arterial blood pressure monitoring* is strongly recommended for the transfer of critically ill patients. Non-invasive blood pressure cuff readings are not able to give a 'real time' view of changes in blood pressure and can be very unreliable. The cuff pressure readings can be corrupted by excessive vibration and non-invasive cuff readings result in a greater drain on the power source. It is more effective to monitor cardiovascular parameters by using invasive pressure lines. Direct arterial and central venous pressure monitoring gives the transfer team immediate information. Transducers should be secured to the patient at an appropriate level since access may be impossible during the transfer (see Chapter 9).

Central venous pressure is measured using the same technology as invasive arterial pressure. If the transport monitor has two invasive pressure channels, both may be displayed en route. If only one is available, arterial monitoring is more valuable.

Urine output measurements should be continued during transfer, using graduated containers for accurate recording. Depending on the length of the transfer, the hourly urine output should be monitored throughout the transfer as a measure of organ (renal) perfusion. Particular attention should be paid to emptying the urine container prior to transferring the patient between the bed and the stretcher; otherwise someone may lay the container flat for the transfer across, losing the current aliquot of urine collected.

Temperature monitoring (e.g. nasopharyngeal, oesophageal, urinary bladder or rectal) should be undertaken in all critical care transfers and considered, together with peripheral temperatures, during transfer.

## Cardiovascular threats

These include cardiac rhythm disturbances, sudden changes in blood pressure and loss of monitoring. It is outside the scope of this book to give a detailed description of the causes and treatment of all the cardiovascular problems that can occur during transfer. However, Table 10.1 demonstrates a logical structure for identifying a few of these potential cardiovascular problems.

| **Table 10.1** Structure for identifying some potential cardiovascular problems | | |
|---|---|---|
| | **Sign** | **Aetiology** |
| Heart rate | Tachycardia | Hypovolaemia<br>Pain/awareness |
| | Bradycardia | Raised intracranial pressure<br>Excessive sedation<br>Hypoxia (neonates and infants) |
| Rhythm | Arrythmias | Electrolyte imbalance/myocardial damage<br>Drug side effects (e.g. aminophyline) |
| Blood pressure | Hypotension | Hypovolaemia<br>Interruption of inotrope infusions |
| | Hypertension | Pain/awareness |

### *Loss of invasive monitor waveforms*

Any invasive line can be blocked with thrombus if not flushed effectively. If a pressure waveform disappears from the screen, the patient should be checked for other signs of clinical deterioration before investigating the monitor.

---

**Actions**

- Check pressure bags are inflated to an appropriate level, or infusion pumps are primed and engaged, and all the connections along the flush line are secure to the transducer
- Check that the transducer will register a pressure rise when the line is flushed manually
- Ensure the cable interface to your monitor is securely connected

---

### *Monitor or syringe pump power failure*

All monitors and pumps can potentially suffer power failure in transit. Replacement batteries can be carried for some models but they may be heavy and require extra space. Older nickel/cadmium batteries often fail to hold charge to the full extent of the quoted duration. Some syringe drivers can operate with conventional dry cell batteries, which are easily inserted. When planning the transfer, consider using a 12 V DC to 240 V AC inverter to allow access to the ambulance battery on transfers. As discussed in Chapter 9 an inverter must be installed by an engineer and used according to instructions in order to ensure safety from electrocution.

---

**Actions**

- Replace batteries if practicable
- Sacrifice a less essential infusion drug and swap syringe drivers
- Use any monitoring resources available in the ambulance
- Resort to basic 'look, listen and feel' monitoring

---

## 10.7 Disability

Rapid changes in acceleration and deceleration forces will result in rises in intracranial pressure (ICP) that can compromise cerebral perfusion. Maintaining a constant speed and minimising sudden turns is therefore beneficial when transferring a patient with a traumatic brain injury. Even if the patient's cervical spine has been cleared radiologically, it is good practice to secure the patient head up and in head blocks to avoid twisting or turning of the head and neck, which impairs venous drainage from an already compromised brain. Limb fractures should be splinted as this can help to reduce pain. Ensure that analgesia is not overlooked in the desire to reduce the number of syringe pumps; local anaesthetic blockade should be considered in the case of rib or limb fractures.

Awareness during transfer is just as frightening as it is in the operating theatre. For children, awareness of strangers in the absence of parents can be terrifying. The possibility of awareness in a child should mandate the inclusion of an accompanying parent unless this is physically impossible.

Despite detailed assessment and resuscitation, occasionally patients undergo a rapid deterioration and die during the transfer. Relatives should never leave the referring centre ahead of the transfer team in order to avoid the possibility of not being available if there is deterioration before departure. The team should be aware of the possibility of deterioration en route and plan accordingly.

The apparently sedated or unconscious patient needs continuing neurological assessment during the transfer. It is embarrassing, to say the least, when staff at the receiving hospital identify a major pupillary change that has not been noted by the transferring team. The position of the eyes and response of the pupils may be the only clinical sign available to confirm elevated ICP. In addition, the only evidence of an underlying convulsion in the paralysed patient may be abnormally responding pupils. A member of the transfer team should be positioned so as to be able to inspect pupillary responses to light. A bright handheld light source should be available for this.

If the ICP is being monitored beforehand, it may be possible to continue this during transfer. Intraparenchymal devices, inserted directly into superficial brain tissue through a small hole drilled in the skull, are commonly used to measure ICP. The ICP monitoring system may have an adequate battery for transfer. Not all neurosurgical centres use the same monitoring devices, so compatibility of equipment after transfer may be an issue affecting whether or not to insert such a monitor immediately prior to transfer. Checking pupillary responses, while clearly less discriminating than ICP, should still be regarded as part of the neurological monitoring during transfer even if an ICP monitor is in use. Ideally, the degree of paralysis as a result of neuromuscular blockade should also be monitored with a nerve stimulator. However, access to limbs may be limited and facial twitches can be difficult to interpret during transit. A detailed description of the monitoring of ICP and neuromuscular blockade is outside the scope of this book.

### Disability threats

Within the disability part of the assessment structure, threats include the failure of the delivery of sedation, analgesia or muscle relaxant drugs (Box 10.7).

> **Box 10.7 Pre-transfer checklist – disability**
>
> - Does the patient require analgesia?
> - Does the patient require sedation?
> - Should the patient be paralysed?
> - Assess the patient's neurological status in the ambulance
> - Plan how the team will respond to changes in the patient's neurological status

Sweating, tachycardia, hypertension and coughing may all be signs that the level of sedation or analgesia is not adequate. It is important to rule out critical problems with the cardiovascular system. To ensure that an ET tube can be tolerated, the patient must be adequately sedated (and paralysed when necessary). Coughing and non-compliance with the ventilator in the presence of a patent ET tube indicate the need to check that sedative and analgesic medications are being delivered.

> **Actions**
>
> - Check the integrity and patency of associated IV lines
> - Check correct functioning of any syringe drivers delivering sedation and analgesia

## 10.8 Exposure and environment

The transporting vehicle can be a hostile place for both patient and transfer personnel. A low ambient temperature may render the unconscious patient hypothermic since a thermo-neutral environment is often difficult to achieve. Body temperature can fall further during the often protracted process of moving to and from vehicles (Box 10.8). This is especially true of children and neonates even when they are being transported in a pod or incubator.

> **Box 10.8 Pre-transfer checklist – exposure and environment**
>
> - Has the patient been kept warm during assessment and stabilisation?
> - Is the patient adequately covered and secured?
> - Is the monitoring and therapeutic equipment adequately secured?
> - Are all personnel going to be adequately secured?

There is a constant threat from unsecured equipment during transfer. It is essential that all equipment is secured or appropriately stored away when not in use. All equipment must be strapped securely to the stretcher/transport trolley or surrounding framework of the ambulance and the stretcher/trolley must, in turn, be secured to the ambulance itself (Box 10.8). All personnel must wear seat belts at all times, unless the vehicle has come to a complete stop. If planning has achieved its aim, then the team should have easy visible and tactile access to all important parts of the patient and monitoring package. Any emergency procedure that will require a team member to leave their seat should only be undertaken when the ambulance is at a standstill.

> **Actions**
>
> - Is emergency clinical intervention required?
> - Can action be undertaken from the seat?
> - Wherever possible, stop the ambulance to deal with the emergency

## 10.9 Arriving at the receiving unit

The arrival and handover procedure should follow the ACCEPT structure, although the order of some of the components may be changed and the concept of evaluation reverts to the normal understanding of the word and its association with reflective practice (Table 10.2).

**Table 10.2** Use of ACCEPT in handover

| ACCEPT | Use in handover |
| --- | --- |
| **A** Assessment | Combine assessment and 'a summary of the transfer process' |
| **C** Control | The handing over of control |
| **C** Communicate | Communicate the 'history of the transfer and the evaluation' |
| **E** Evaluate | Reflect on the whole of the transfer process |
| **P** Prepare and package | Unpack the patient |
| **T** Transportation | Transfer the patient |

Before arriving at the recipient unit, mentally repeat the steps undertaken during the original assessment. Remember the 'soundbite' and the systematic approach to the problems and the actions taken. The team should be in a position to reflect on the transfer and to make a general evaluation as to their satisfaction with the process so far. This reflection on assessment and ongoing evaluation should inform the team of an appropriate structure to communicate a potentially complex story in a concise, logical and clear fashion.

While the transferring team leader is still in control, there is a need to agree when the receiving unit's team leader will take over. In most cases, the unspoken agreement is that a full multi-disciplinary handover should occur first. After this, the patient should be transferred to the receiving unit bed and attached to the receiving unit ventilator. Until this point is reached the transferring team remain in overall charge. There is then a 'grey area', during which monitoring and syringe driver medications are transferred to the receiving unit's equipment.

Prepare and package now becomes prepare to unpackage. A systematic plan for attaching the patient to the receiving unit's equipment should be agreed.

Unpacking, and executing the actual transfer of the patient, requires team work. The whole procedure should be discussed and a plan formulated and executed under the control of one or other team leaders. Special care needs to be taken during this transfer to ensure that tubes, drains and lines are not dislodged during the move from the trolley or incubator to the intensive care unit cot or bed. One example of assessing risk is shown in Box 10.9.

---

### Box 10.9 Example of risk assessment

The **assessment** shows there is a significant risk of ET tube dislodgement during the transfer from stretcher to bed

The **plan** might be:

- Check that the ET tube is still secure
- Check that the level of the tube at the lips has not changed from the recorded value
- Check that the patient is receiving 100% oxygen
- Allocate a team member to hold the ET tube
- Consider disconnecting the patient from the breathing circuit for the period of the move
- Consider not disconnecting but ensure that the breathing circuit is not going to drag on the ET tube

---

### Implementation of the plan

Once everyone involved is briefed and the team leader agrees then the plan is executed.

Before returning to the base hospital, the transfer team should ensure that they have handed over all the case notes, X-rays and laboratory investigations. Many hospitals now collect data on inter-hospital transfers and submit these data to national audits such as ICBIS (Intensive Care Bed Information Service) or PICANET (Paediatric Intensive Care Audit Network); these forms must be completed and returned to the appropriate place.

Checks should ensure that all medical equipment is cleaned, decontaminated and returned appropriately. Any equipment thought to be faulty should be quarantined and a clear history of the circumstances around the problem should be given to the electrical or biomedical engineers. Any partially used sedation syringes or other unused drugs must be securely disposed of before returning to the ambulance. The mnemonic **CLEAR** can be used as an aide-mémoire.

---

**CLEAR**

**C** Case notes and radiographs
**L** Laboratory investigations
**E** Evaluation (as reflective process)
**A** Audit form or transfer record
**R** Return equipment and dispose of drugs

---

## 10.10 Summary

Attention to detail at all three stages of the transfer will ensure that the patient is delivered in the best possible condition.

PART 3
# Practical considerations

# CHAPTER 11

# SCRUMP – the differences between transport and hospital-based care

---

### Learning outcomes

After reading this, you will be able to:
- Discuss the key differences between transport medicine and hospital-based care
- Identify key considerations that should be addressed before moving a patient

---

## 11.1 Introduction

As soon as the decision is taken to move a patient from one clinical environment to another, staff involved need to plan to ensure the journey is undertaken carefully, safely and without undue risk. When the move is from one hospital to another some of the issues are clear and immediate and often predominate any plan: Who will accompany the patient? What means of transport should be used? How urgent is the transfer? Too often these are the only issues that are considered, resulting in a transfer process that may leave practitioners exposed, working in an unfamiliar environment with equipment they are unaccustomed to using, travelling at unsafe speeds and with a patient or equipment that is inadequately secured.

This chapter aims to discuss in more detail the SCRUMP acronym that was introduced in Chapter 2. SCRUMP aims to provide a quick mental checklist of key issues that should be considered before undertaking any transfer:

| | |
|---|---|
| **S** | Shared assessment |
| **C** | Clinical isolation |
| **R** | Resource limitation |
| **U** | Unfamiliar equipment |
| **M** | Movement and safety |
| **P** | Physical and physiological changes |

The focus of this chapter is on the transportation of patients between hospitals. However, the same approach can, and should, be applied in other situations: for example the move of a patient from the emergency department to a ward bed, or from a hospital ward to the radiology department for a scan. In every case use of the SCRUMP acronym will help to ensure that the staff involved in moving the patient have communicated clearly between the referring and receiving care areas, decided who should accompany the patient, considered equipment familiarity and the best means of transport.

---

*Neonatal, Adult and Paediatric Safe Transfer and Retrieval: A Practical Approach to Transfers*, First Edition.
Edited by Bernard Foëx, Peter-Marc Fortune and Cassie Lawn.
© 2019 John Wiley & Sons Ltd. Published 2019 by John Wiley & Sons Ltd.

## 11.2  Shared assessment

Whenever a patient is to be moved from one hospital to another, information about their clinical condition and the need for transfer is exchanged between the referring and receiving clinical teams. The ACCEPT principles outlined in Chapters 5–9 provide a clear structure by which clinicians can ensure the referral is thorough and systematic (Box 11.1).

### Box 11.1  The SCRUMP and ACCEPT mnemonics

| S  Shared assessment | A  Assessment | What is the problem? (think summary)<br>What is being done? (think background)<br>What is the effect? (think assessment)<br>What is needed now? (think recommendation) | |
|---|---|---|---|
| | C  Control | Identify team leader(s)<br>• Clinical<br>• Logistic<br>Identify and allocate tasks to be carried out<br>Pre-transport advice: ABCDEF | |
| | C  Communication | Communication – what:<br>• Who you are -contact details<br>• What the problem is (soundbite)<br>• Relevant details<br>• What you need from the listener<br>• What you have done<br>• Effect of these actions<br>• Summarise agreed plans<br>• What you need from the listener | Communication – with who:<br>• Local team<br>• Transfer team<br>• Receiving team<br>• Ambulance control<br>• Family |
| | E  Evaluation | Establish urgency of transfer<br>Is the transfer appropriate – going to the right place?<br>Speed and mode of transfer | |
| C  Clinical isolation<br>R  Resource limitation<br>U  Unfamiliar equipment<br>M  Movement and safety<br>P  Physical and physiological changes | P  Preparation<br>P  Packaging<br>P  Pre-departure checks | Checks of patient, equipment and personnel | |
| | T  Transportation | Handover – CLEAR | |

What remains key to the process is an agreed assessment of clinical priorities; subsequent decision making is based on that assessment. A neurosurgeon may advise that a patient is transferred 'as quickly as possible'; a radiographer may suggest that a patient is brought to the scanner immediately; a receiving intensive care unit may suggest that it is safe for a patient to remain locally for a number of hours before they are transferred. In each instance it is vital that enough clinical information is shared so that the patient can be managed in the referring centre, and so the transport episode can be undertaken with appropriate staff, equipment and monitoring.

Key to the assessment process is developing the ability to accurately describe a clinical situation and to convey enough relevant information such that the receiver can form an image of the patient, their illness and the available resources. Tools such as SBAR (situation, background, assessment and recommendation) (NHS Improvement, 2018) are an excellent starting point for conveying information rapidly and in a structured way when an immediate response is required, but may provide insufficient information when planning to move a critically ill patient. Almost certainly the clinician undertaking the transfer will need to ask questions to complete their picture of the patient. Referrers should expect the referral process to be interactive, rather than an exercise in direct transmission. The whole referral process should result in clarity and understanding as to the next steps for both parties.

There are several ways in which the process of referral may be enhanced to ensure clear communication.

## Standardised forms

All transport services use their own standardised form to collect referral information. An example of one such form is included in Appendix D. Many services also make a version of the form available to referring centres. This has the advantage of clearly laying out the information in an agreed format, smoothing communication between referrer and receiver. If a referring centre can spend a few moments gathering relevant clinical and demographic information before calling, the whole process will become more effective.

## Call conferencing/recording

No referrer wants to have to go through the clinical history several times before a decision regarding transport is made. The ability to involve junior and senior staff, as well as to gather specialist opinions during one call is beneficial to all. This may best be achieved by conferencing all parties into a referral call whenever possible. Clearly this is more difficult for ad hoc emergency transfers but has become a required standard of care for paediatric transport services. The NHS England Service Specification for Paediatric Critical Care Transport now states 'there will be a single point of contact through which the PCC Transport Service can be contacted and activated at all times for clinical advice and transport planning. This will include teleconferencing, call handling and call recording functionality' (NHS England E07/S/d, 2015).

## Telemetry

As technology progresses the ability to share clinical data remotely increases. Sophisticated systems exist to share clinical information whilst ensuring data security and confidentiality; transmission of images, X-rays and monitored data may all enhance the referral process.

## Documentation

It is vitally important that the conversation between referrer and receiver is documented, including any advice given and a record of the next agreed management steps. Again, the requirement for paediatric critical care teams is that they install call recording functionality and that clear, accurate and retrievable records of communications are kept (NHS England E07/S/d, 2015).

## 11.3 Clinical isolation

Whenever a patient is moved from one location to another, they are at their most vulnerable during the period of transportation. Apart from the objective aspects of travelling at speed, for staff, this represents the time that they are physically separated from their usual support structures within the hospital. Surprisingly, for many clinicians, the realisation that they are literally 'on their own' only happens once the ambulance doors are closed and an issue develops with either the patient's physiology or with the transport kit. It is essential that everything possible is done to lessen the impact of this period of relative isolation.

Some of the ways clinical isolation may be addressed are listed here.

### Specific transport training and competency assessments

Transport team members should be trained not only in the use of the medical devices (see Section 11.5), but also in the processes underlying safe medical practice. Good training before being asked to transport a patient 'solo' will minimise any sense of unfamiliarity. Many transport teams will have written competency assessments in place to ensure all clinical staff have the necessary level of understanding before embarking on an inter-hospital transfer.

### Experienced and qualified dedicated nursing staff

Because of the nature of medical training, most junior doctors will have limited exposure to working in the transport environment, usually as part of a more general rotation. It stands to reason that they will have less experience in that environment than permanent members of the nursing staff. Within transport medicine, team working is vital and indispensable. By investing in the training and expertise of nursing staff, teams are indirectly providing the most immediate support to medical staff.

## Use of local resources

The sense that a patient is wholly the responsibility of the transferring medical team can be lessened by an explicit encouragement to use local resources wherever possible. Acknowledging that once in an ambulance or aircraft help is hard to come by, it makes sense for teams to use the skills and expertise available in the referring centre should the situation demand. This may involve asking for senior local help – for example when intubating a patient or establishing vascular access – especially when this is difficult or the patient is unstable.

## Telephony

Clinical isolation during the actual transport episode can best be overcome by ensuring rapid, direct telephone support from senior staff is available. It is worth noting that on long motorway journeys standard mobile phone networks may have patchy coverage, especially in more rural areas. Some thought should be given to ensuring that mobile phones using a variety of networks are available, and that, if no coverage is obtainable, the ambulance is fitted with a radio communication system.

## Senior staff

Perhaps the most obvious way of providing direct support to transport team members is to provide senior support within the vehicle. Supervised transfers are the only way of ensuring that teams are supported when caring for the most critically ill patients, and ensure that good working practices are developed and maintained. Frequently, especially when a transfer is being organised ad hoc, either a consultant or a middle grade doctor will accompany a patient, but rarely both. This is one of the aspects of transport medicine that makes training and supervision uniquely difficult. However, centralised transport services are often staffed in such a way that direct supervision is possible, until a new medical team member has achieved familiarity with the transport process or whenever the acuity of the patient's illness demands senior input.

## Emergency back-up

In rare circumstances a transport team may get into difficulty either before departure or during the transport episode. In such circumstances the safety of the patient is paramount and it may be necessary to rapidly dispatch a second relief vehicle with staff who can assist in the stabilisation and transfer of the patient.

## 11.4  Resource limitation

All health care practitioners are used to working in a well-stocked hospital environment, where equipment, medicines and staff are available. Conversely, transport practitioners are limited in the resources they can draw upon – limited by what they have chosen to take with them; limited by what they are physically able to carry; and limited by accessibility to their kit within the ambulance or aircraft. Necessarily, medical equipment will be carried in limited supply, but experience has shown that the most common transport incidents are caused by loss of medical gas supply, loss of electrical power and by vehicular failure (including running out of fuel!). Such losses are, in the main, preventable by careful planning and husbandry of resources.

### Medical gases

#### *Oxygen*

Almost all transports of critically ill patients will rely on the use of oxygen, either via a face mask or to drive a ventilator. Within hospitals, oxygen appears to be essentially limitless – oxygen outlets are provided in high dependency and critical areas although they are, ultimately, supplied from an industrial-sized oxygen container. During transport, the considerations are different. A number of reports have described the morbidity associated with having an inadequate number of oxygen cylinders during transport. There are also published normograms that allow team members to quickly estimate the oxygen required for a journey of given duration. Other services have developed electronic systems to perform the same task. Whichever method is used, the golden rule of transport medicine is to perform this estimate and then to take twice as much as you have calculated you will need, in case of necessity. Regular transport practitioners are also assiduous in ensuring that they preserve their bottled oxygen supplies wherever possible, always choosing to use the hospital supply apart from during the actual transport episode itself.

Most transport ventilators in common use are mechanical, relying on the driving pressure of an oxygen cylinder to function. Having calculated oxygen demand, it is also important to note that the total volume of oxygen taken may well be divided between a number of cylinders. There is nothing worse than a patient becoming desaturated during a transport because the ventilator has stopped working because there is insufficient driving pressure in the attached oxygen cylinder. Responding at this late stage is poor practice, particularly as the event is wholly preventable. One simple method of ensuring a cylinder does not become exhausted is to include a note of the cylinder contents dial with other regular patient observations during the time of transport.

Finally, it is important to ensure that vehicle oxygen supplies are maintained. It is good practice to make a note of the oxygen available when entering an ambulance – not only the cylinder sizes, but also ensuring that the cylinders are full. If there is any concern that there is an insufficient supply, the cylinders should be changed before departing. This may mean taking a patient out of an ambulance to the safety of the hospital oxygen supply while another cylinder is sourced. At the end of a transport episode, systems should be in place to ensure that vehicle oxygen supplies are replenished.

### *Medical air*

The use of medical air for ventilation is primarily in small infants, especially those with complex cardiac abnormalities. All the considerations given above with regard to carefully managing oxygen resources pertain to air as well, with one additional point to bear in mind – bottled medical air is *much* harder to come by than oxygen cylinders and it is crucial that supplies are maintained at all costs. It may prove very difficult to source a replacement medical air cylinder in a hospital that does not have a routine use for them.

### Electrical power

This is the other common resource that can easily run out. It is easy for the unwary practitioner to attach a patient to a vital signs monitor and infusion pumps, without giving due consideration to the fact that they are running on battery power. If the stabilisation and transfer times are prolonged it is possible for all monitoring to be lost as the batteries fail.

As with medical gas supplies, the careful practitioner will ensure that at all possible opportunities their equipment is plugged in and charging. This should include the time before it is used, and any time whilst the patient is being stabilised in the referring centre. Obviously, while the patient is being moved between hospital and ambulance the equipment will have to rely on stored charge, but the majority of modern ambulances will have an electrical management system, and may well be fitted with a power inverter that converts 12 V DC battery power to 240 V AC power. This will allow equipment to be plugged in using a standard three point socket.

The same considerations do *not* apply in flight. In the majority of aircraft there is no opportunity to plug in medical equipment: it is therefore even more crucial to ensure pumps and monitors are fully charged with sufficient reserve to last the journey. Minimising power-hungry functions – particularly non-invasive blood pressure measurements – will help to reduce battery usage.

## 11.5 Unfamiliar equipment

In most cases the equipment that is used in the transport environment is different from that in use within a hospital setting. Monitors, defibrillators, saturation probes, glucometers, syringe drivers, ventilators and blood gas analysers will all be chosen for their transport characteristics – the need to be portable, robust, reliable and capable of being battery driven. All of which may mean that they are less sophisticated than the equivalent equipment used in hospitals.

It is essential that all those involved in transporting patients are not only able to use the supplied equipment safely, but can troubleshoot devices if they do not operate in the expected manner. A system of equipment competency-based training is essential to ensure that patient safety is maintained during transport. Practitioners should be expected to demonstrate that they can set up and use all the necessary equipment; that they have a working understanding of common functions; and they know how to set appropriate alarm limits and to respond to them.

Often doctors will assume that their experienced nursing colleague will be able to operate the equipment and to troubleshoot any problems that arise. Whilst this is generally true, it does not make for safe practice. It is also remarkably inefficient – team working can only be at its best when both medical and nursing staff are able to work together.

## 11.6 Movement and safety

Perhaps the most obvious difference between hospital-based practice and transport medicine is the fact that the patient and staff are physically moving. UK accident data show several hundred incidents involving ambulances each year, frequently resulting in serious injury and occasionally in fatalities. Moreover, analysis of ambulance accident data from the USA shows that when ambulances are involved in a collision, it is the personnel in the rear cabin who are the most vulnerable. In ambulance crashes resulting in a fatality, 72% of deaths occurred in personnel riding in the ambulance rear cabin and, within this group, 73% were unrestrained at the time of the incident. These facts have lead European legislators to insist that all modern ambulances are fitted with seats and harnesses that meet safety legislation – but they can only perform their function if they are worn. Often in the past, clinicians would undo their seatbelt to attend to their patient or a piece of equipment; it was not uncommon for staff to walk around the rear cabin in search of an otherwise inaccessible drug or syringe, all while the ambulance was moving at speed. This is completely unacceptable. Whenever a team member needs to leave their seat, the driver should be asked to slow and stop the vehicle as soon as it is safe to do so and only then should staff in the rear cabin undo their seatbelts and move about. All these issues are more fully dealt with in Chapter 12.

European CEN regulations also insist that equipment in an ambulance should be secured and capable of withstanding a crash at 30 mph (in any direction, assuming an abrupt stop). Table 11.1 assumes a head-on crash with abrupt deceleration.

At a speed of 30 mph the G-force is 10 g. An unsecured 5 kg ventilator will therefore act as a 50 kg object when travelling at that speed. An unsecured team member will exert a force equivalent to more than half a ton. It is vital that everything in the back of an ambulance, including the patient, equipment and staff, are restrained adequately. Any equipment not required during the journey should be safely stowed.

| Table 11.1 Speed and G-force in a head-on crash | |
| --- | --- |
| **Speed (mph)** | **G-force (g)** |
| 30 | 10 |
| 40 | 17 |
| 60 | 24 |
| 100 | 40 |

## 11.7 Physical and physiological changes

The cold, dark, noisy, vibrating environment of an ambulance cabin provides specific challenges to any team moving a patient.

### Thermoregulation

This is an issue for all patients, where there may be a conflict between a desire to keep a patient under close observation versus the need to keep them warm; however it is particularly true of neonates and small infants who have a high ratio of surface area to volume and poor thermoregulatory homeostatic mechanisms. Ideally, the rear cabin of an ambulance will have electronic climate control, enabling staff to control the ambient temperature. Teams need to carry a variety of warming devices to ensure good thermoregulation, including chemically activated gel mattresses (Transwarmer™), blankets and foil blankets.

### Vision

Ambulances can be dark and can vibrate, both of which circumstances can make assessing a patient or reading a pump or monitor more difficult. Crucially, however, it is the constraint of space and consequent poor lines of sight that makes vision difficult. Time spent assessing where equipment and personnel will be placed is well spent. Where monitors cannot be seen easily, it is crucial to ensure that any alarm is set with an auditory component and that the volume is set loudly enough to be heard above any associated road noise/sirens.

**Flight**

There are many specific physiological changes associated with flight. These are dealt with in Chapter 17.

## 11.8 Summary

There are specific considerations to be taken into account before undertaking any patient transfer, beyond the initial considerations of who will take them and how will they travel.

The SCRUMP mnemonic provides a useful way of remembering six key issues that affect any transfer.

- **S**hared assessment
- **C**linical isolation
- **R**esource limitation
- **U**nfamiliar equipment
- **M**ovement and safety
- **P**hysical and physiological changes

Ensuring that these have been well thought through before transporting a patient will help ensure best practice.

# CHAPTER 12
# Safety and the team

---

## Learning outcomes

After reading this, you will be able to:
- Describe the importance of keeping the clinical team safe during transfer
- Explain the importance of keeping the patient and carers safe during a transfer
- Discuss how to minimise risks to safety from an organisational perspective

---

## 12.1 Introduction

Safely transporting a critically ill patient requires a coordinated approach. The transport environment is hazardous. Travelling in the rear compartment of a road ambulance or aircraft is fraught with potential danger.

Safety is one of the basic domains of healthcare standards that govern the operation of NHS trusts and is guided by legislation. Health and safety at work regulations have several specific provisions which are pertinent to the field of transfer medicine, and include the following:

- Management of Health and Safety at Work Regulations 1999 (management regulations that cover general duty of care to ensure the safety of staff, and others, on an employer's premises). Patients are included under 'others'
- Manual Handling Operations Regulations 2002
- Personal Protective Equipment at Work Regulations 1992
- Control of Substances Hazardous to Health Regulations 2002
- Noise at Work Regulations 1989

This chapter will focus on safety in the transport environment (Figure 12.1) in terms of:

- The team
- The patient
- The carers
- The vehicle and equipment
- The organisation

## 12.2 The team

### Clothing

All staff should prepare for the worst. It is never possible to predict whether an ambulance is likely to break down or be involved in an incident, therefore adequate clothing should always be carried to ensure sufficient protection against the weather. Proprietary reflective jackets or vests should be provided for all staff to ensure good visibility if they have to step outside the ambulance whilst parked at the roadside. Shoes should afford maximum protection from equipment incidents and be appropriate for the roadside environment; theatre clogs are not suitable for undertaking external transfers.

---

*Neonatal, Adult and Paediatric Safe Transfer and Retrieval: A Practical Approach to Transfers*, First Edition.
Edited by Bernard Foëx, Peter-Marc Fortune and Cassie Lawn.
© 2019 John Wiley & Sons Ltd. Published 2019 by John Wiley & Sons Ltd.

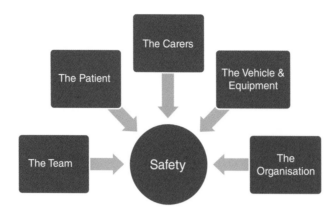

**Figure 12.1 Elements of transport safety**

## Manual handling

Musculoskeletal disorders account for approximately 40% of all sickness absence in the NHS. Nurses are known to have a high rate of musculoskeletal disorders; ambulance staff have an even higher rate of sickness, due to back injury. Over 80% of ill health retirements from the ambulance service are due to back injury and musculoskeletal disorders. It is a requirement that all staff should receive moving and handling training with team members, ensuring that all manual handling activities are in line with legislation as detailed in the Health and Safety at Work Act 1974 and the Manual Handling Operations Regulations 1992 (as amended 2004) (MHOR) and local policy. Medical staff are not excluded.

Transfers are often undertaken in cramped conditions and may involve movement of heavy patients and equipment into and out of ambulances and other vehicles. These movements present a significant risk to the health of transfer personnel. A risk assessment by your trust manual handling services may identify some useful ways of reducing this risk. Whether or not this is undertaken, each team member is responsible for assessing the risks both to themselves and others.

Where possible, automated equipment should be used (e.g. tail lifts) to load patient stretchers and equipment bags with loose equipment packed into specially designed trolleys/bags and stowed securely. If these facilities are not available, use stretcher trolleys or wheelchairs with appropriate safety straps to transport equipment. Do not hesitate to ask for help from local staff when required.

Established teams should examine their transport kit and pursue modifications that may improve manual handling characteristics. Always use a Patslide™ or other appropriate aid to move patients between stretchers.

Be careful: the transport environment is not kind to backs!

## Infection control

All team members should be fully immunised against hepatitis B. Never compromise on the use of standard precautions. Hand hygiene should not be forgotten and personal protective equipment (PPE) should always be used as it would be on the ward.

It is best practice to always assume that the patient is infectious and behave accordingly, as it is uncommon for microbiology results to be available before the departure of the transport team.

Be especially careful with bodily fluids, including respiratory secretions when intubating and suctioning. Always wear a surgical mask and eye protection, or use a closed system.

Where there is a suspicion of an especially virulent and highly infectious pathogen, special precautions must be taken. These include double gloving/gown/goggles/N95 mask or filtering face piece respirator (FFP3) or powered air-purifying respirator (PAPR) as appropriate and as guided by local policy. Only those trained and regularly updated in their use should wear these types of PPE. For further information, consult the Health Protection Agency (www.hpa.org.uk) or local microbiology service.

## Sharps

The potential to sustain a sharps injury during the resuscitation and stabilisation of a critically ill patient, in unfamiliar territory, such as another hospital or the back of an ambulance, is higher than in a practitioner's usual place of work. Be extra vigilant. Find out where the sharps bin is and ensure that your sharps are immediately disposed of. Be watchful of others and do not injure yourself on someone else's sharps.

Ensure that the transfer vehicle you use has an easily accessible sharps bin. All syringes that are preloaded for the journey should be capped off with needleless caps, not sheathed syringe needles.

## Restraint

All staff travelling in an ambulance or other vehicle must wear seatbelts whilst the vehicle is in motion. If interventions are required that cannot be performed by a team member in the seated, belted position, the vehicle must be stopped, ensuring that it is done in a safe manner.

Wherever possible, team members should be seated such that they have access to the patient and an adequate view of the monitors. Access to infusion pumps and infusion lines for giving fluid boluses should also be possible.

An unrestrained team member becomes a missile in a collision.

## 12.3 The patient

### Clothing

Heat loss through convection, conduction and radiation are all increased in the transfer environment. Careful wrapping of the patient to minimise heat loss, without compromising access for clinical observations and interventions, can be very difficult. The use of foil thermal wraps, vacuum mattresses and the BabyPODII™ (in the case of infants up to 5 kg) can all help in this regard. If using a vacuum mattress with a heating gel pack, small patients may become overheated. The patient's temperature should be measured continuously.

Where a patient is fully anaesthetised, exposure when moving between vehicles may be minimised by completely covering them for a brief time. If you do use this method it is important to be explicit about your intentions to ensure that nobody interprets the covering as signal of death!

### Infection control

Critically ill patients may have impaired immunity. It is important not to compromise on sterile technique when inserting or accessing lines, drains or catheters during a transfer.

Hand hygiene should not be forgotten and PPE should always be used as it would be on the ward.

### Restraint

Over the body 'cross-straps' provided as standard on most ambulance stretchers provide very little restraint in the horizontal plane. Currently, commercially available 'over the shoulder', adjustable, five-point harnesses are not available for all sizes of patient. There is therefore no definitive solution at the moment. A number of companies have done work in this area for smaller patients with products such as the ACR™ (Figure 12.2) and Pedimate™ being useful solutions for patients weighing between 5 and 45 kg (Pedimate up to 15 kg). For neonatal patients in incubators and for larger patients, NeoRestraint™ 'over the shoulder' trolley straps (Figure 12.3) are preferable to 'cross-straps'.

(a)

(b)

(c)

(d)

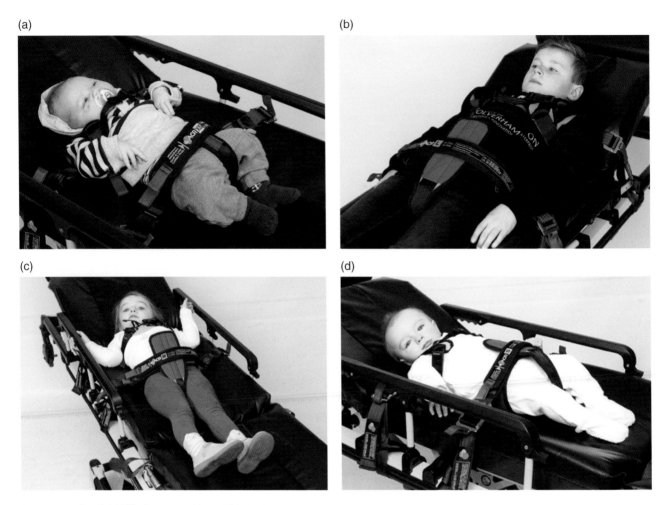

**Figure 12.2 (a–d) ACR™.** Courtesy of ParAid Medical

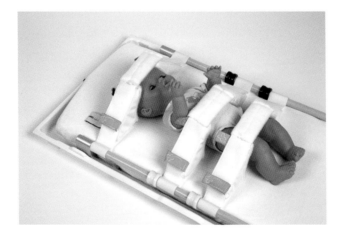

**Figure 12.3 NeoRestraint™.** Courtesy of ParAid Medical

## 12.4 The carers

### Clothing

If carers accompany the transport team it is important that they have appropriate clothing and footwear for all eventualities as described above for the staff.

## Restraint

When travelling in the ambulance, family must always wear the seatbelt provided. It must be made clear that they must not release it unless the ambulance has come to a halt and the transport team and/or driver instruct them that it is safe to do so.

# 12.5 The vehicle and equipment

### Equipment and manual handling

General issues of manual handling are discussed earlier in this chapter. Equipment should be assembled into bags or boxes, which ideally wheel along but may be carried if that is not possible. As before, your trust manual handling department may be helpful with the design of kit that meets the needs of the team with minimisation of manual handling risk.

### Infection control

All equipment should be clean and uncontaminated. Use breathing system filters to protect the patient and the ventilator. An appropriate maintenance/cleaning schedule for all equipment should be adhered to.

### Restraint

Unrestrained equipment becomes a missile when sudden deceleration occurs during a collision. All equipment, no matter how small and insignificant, must be restrained. Established retrieval teams should ensure that it is possible to secure all of their equipment into the back of the ambulance, in compliance with CEN guidelines (see next section).

For ad hoc teams a compromise using over the top 'cross-straps' on the ambulance stretcher may be useful to restrain equipment; however, it should be remembered that such straps provide very little restraint in the horizontal plane. Most ambulances also have appropriate restraints for portable oxygen bottles, but, if not, make sure they are put away in cupboards or strapped down firmly elsewhere. Cupboard space should also be used for all other loose items of equipment.

### Ambulance

The CEN (European Committee for Standardisation) standard for ambulances in the UK (BS EN 1789:2007 – Medical vehicles and their equipment – Road ambulances) is voluntary. The Vehicle Certification Agency (www.vca.gov.uk) provides certificates of CEN compliance, and most ambulance providers are ensuring that newly purchased vehicles are CEN certified.

It is notable that equipment not normally carried in the ambulance is exempt from this regulation, and also the restraint of patients in the rear compartment of the ambulance is not regulated. Despite this, everyone involved in transfers should seek the best possible solutions for both their own and the patient's safety.

### Manual handling

Ambulance crews are used to manual handling and are a useful resource. Hydraulic lifts should be used wherever provided to load and unload stretchers, incubators, equipment and bags.

For stability, height adjustable stretchers should only be moved when at their lowest position to prevent tipping – this means that extendable handles need to be used to manoeuvre the stretcher.

### Infection control

Cleaning schedules for ambulance interiors should be adhered to and documented as suggested by the Joint Royal Colleges Ambulance Liaison Committee (JRCALC).

### Sharps

A sharps bin should be available in the ambulance – make sure it is within reach if it is required during the journey.

### Restraint

All passengers must use seatbelt restraints where fitted – preferably a full three-point harness. No one should stand up whilst the ambulance is moving – always ask the driver to stop in a safe place first.

When you board the vehicle have a look at the interior and note the position of the fixtures and fittings. If anyone is unrestrained in the rear of the ambulance, they may become a missile, and the projecting fittings are areas with which they will collide. Other occupants will also be endangered by an unrestrained passenger. Think about where staff sit – if you are unable to restrain the patient adequately, the rearward facing seat at the patient's head should only be used if there is no alternative.

If you are fortunate enough to have a purpose-built vehicle for transfers, make sure that the cupboards can be used to store your equipment and that there are clamps for all equipment necessary for transfer (trolley/ventilator/pumps, etc.).

## Speed

There is often a sense of urgency about transport of the critically ill patient. This may lead to the use of lights and sirens and emergency driving techniques on both outbound and inbound journeys. There is evidence that very little time is saved, and the risks of collision are increased during journeys where lights and sirens and exemptions (such as speeding and passing through red lights) are used.

The acceleration and deceleration forces associated with this sort of driving technique are increased and may affect the team in terms of their comfort and ability to perform their duties. On the return journey, the patient may be compromised by such driving due to potentially reduced physiological stability. This is especially true in the preterm infant and cardiovascularly unstable patient.

Travelling using lights and sirens and exemptions over long distances is more stressful and tiring for the driver and may be harmful for the patient. For all these reasons, emergency driving techniques are not normally necessary or desirable.

Strategies to reduce the need for emergency driving techniques include the following:

- Promote a culture of safety over speed
- Use telephone advice to support local resources in the resuscitation and stabilisation of the critically ill patient
- Reduce transport team mobilisation time
- Ensure that the destination and route is confirmed prior to departure
- Prepare the patient for stable transfer
- Pursue a system of smooth progress with the traffic
- Use clinical triage to stratify urgency and inform driving techniques. For example, categorise a journey from 1 to 3 (Table 12.1). Ambulance technicians undergo training that translates the clinical category into driving behaviour. They retain the responsibility for the use or otherwise of emergency driving techniques and exemptions. Medical and nursing staff therefore should make no judgement of the driving technique that may be required on the journey (for which they are not trained) and do not dictate the use of exemptions

| Table 12.1 Categories of journey | | |
|---|---|---|
| **Category 1** | **Category 2** | **Category 3** |
| Emergency call | Emergency call | Non-emergency call |
| Requires a blue light response | Predetermined times are set by transport team to travel to and from referring hospitals | No need to use exemptions |
| | Exemptions should be used if these predetermined times will be exceeded without exemptions | |

Convoys of blue light vehicles are more dangerous than a single vehicle, with the second vehicle being the most vulnerable – for this reason, in some parts of the country, the police do not provide police escorts to ambulances.

Do not use excessive speed or cross red lights unless absolutely necessary. The use of exemptions should only be considered under exceptional circumstances.

## 12.6 The organisation

### Operational and clinical protocols

A culture that promotes safety and team working must exist to allow the highest quality and safest care to be delivered.

Standard operating procedures (SOPs) are generally established from evidence-based best practices and guide the procedures so they are carried out in the same way to the same standard irrespective of the individual carrying them out. They can range from administrative and logistical to medical and nursing.

Some regard SOPs as unnecessarily binding and that, particularly with clinical SOPs, the practitioner should be free to deviate from the protocol according to their professional judgement. However, they are a useful tool for the transport team to ensure that the care delivery remains focused and safe throughout the process.

### Clinical governance and audit

Clinical governance provides a structure to ensure that high quality care is delivered and is discussed in detail in Chapter 21.

### Checklists

Checklists are usually an extension of an SOP. They are lists of jobs or tasks that need to be done, usually in a particular order, with a list of points to remember and they serve as aides-memoires.

Checklists are used in many fields, from health and safety inspections and machinery functional checks to complex aircraft emergency procedures and surgical procedures. They should be relevant to the task to be performed and should contain sufficient detail without becoming laborious.

The use of well organised and appropriate checklists in the transport environment can aid team/practitioner performance, contribute to care quality and risk management.

### Team training

All practitioners involved in transfers must be appropriately trained. They must be able to demonstrate their competence not only in intensive care medicine/nursing but also their ability to deliver this in the transport environment. Trusts with designated transport services should provide specific transport training, relating it to local guidelines and equipment.

Team training should also include training for non-technical skills (NTS) such as human factors and team resource management (TRM). Teams with highly developed NTS will have improved performance and reduced risk.

Competency documents should be used and reviewed on a yearly basis.

### Insurance

All NHS staff are entitled to benefit from the NHS Injury Benefits Scheme. Within a trust the chief executive carries responsibility for the maintenance of all standards within the trust and is ultimately responsible for the actions and omissions of all staff employed by the trust. This is known as vicarious liability. This and insurance requirements for transport teams are discussed in detail in Chapter 21.

## 12.7 Summary

The transport of the critically ill patient aims to provide safe transfer from the referring to receiving centre. This requires a multi-disciplinary approach to all aspects of service provision, with an emphasis on a culture of safety.

Single interventions are unlikely to have a significant effect in improving safety, but an approach that builds a culture of safety throughout the service should be linked to significant improvements in care delivery.

# PART 4
# Clinical considerations

This section will focus on the assessment and treatment of a patient requiring a transfer to facilitate either ongoing care or clinical investigations.

Chapter 13 provides a generic overview: the key steps that should be followed for all patients are the same irrespective of gestation, age or diagnosis. The process of continual, ongoing assessment and planning is also agnostic of patient type and will be illustrated throughout.

The following chapters that make up this section provide a discussion of the most common problems specific to each of the relevant age groups (neonates, children and adults). It is important to note that these chapters only provide an overview; a more in-depth description of pathophysiological processes and definitive treatments are outside the scope of this book.

# CHAPTER 13
# Clinical considerations – an introduction

---

**Learning outcomes**

After reading this chapter, you will be able to:
- Identify the structured approach to the clinical assessment and initial care of a patient requiring transfer, using the ABCDEF approach to structure primary and secondary surveys
- Outline the utility of a primary, simplified clinical assessment before proceeding to more complex and comprehensive methods of assessment

---

## 13.1 Introduction

The primary survey (for infants this is called the initial approach assessment and stabilisation of any potentially life-threatening problems) followed by the secondary survey (for infants called the reassessment and planning of definitive care) are outlined in this chapter.

In hospitalised patients this is best delivered using a recognised structured approach. This has the advantage of being successfully reproducible, with the minimum of omissions or errors in stressful situations. It also presents a method that is recognised by the whole of the multi-disciplinary team, which assists in the smooth functioning of that team. This is especially true of ad hoc resuscitation teams who may not know one another. The ABCDEF structure is an internationally recognised approach and should be used for this purpose. It is universally applicable to all scenarios and age groups. Its application is described in detail in the Neonatal Life Support (NLS), Advanced Resuscitation of the Newborn Infant (ARNI), Advanced Paediatric Life Support (APLS), Advanced Life Support (ALS) and Advanced Trauma Life Support (ATLS) manuals and their associated courses. The structure is summarised in Box 13.1.

---

**Box 13.1 ABCDEF approach**

**A**  Airway assessment and control
**B**  Breathing
**C**  Circulation
**D**  Disability and Dextrose
**E**  Exposure (including temperature in neonates and children) and Everything else
**F**  Family

---

A rapid assessment of ABC is undertaken first and problems are addressed as they are identified, followed by a more detailed examination; i.e. primary survey followed by secondary survey. This approach is used to underpin the care delivered throughout the treat and transfer process.

---

*Neonatal, Adult and Paediatric Safe Transfer and Retrieval: A Practical Approach to Transfers*, First Edition.
Edited by Bernard Foëx, Peter-Marc Fortune and Cassie Lawn.
© 2019 John Wiley & Sons Ltd. Published 2019 by John Wiley & Sons Ltd.

## 13.2 Initial assessment and stabilisation

> *Rapidly seek out and **treat** all immediately life-threatening conditions.*

The aim of the primary survey is to identify and treat any immediately life-threatening conditions (Table 13.1). This differs from traditional clinical teaching of taking a history from the patient followed by clinical examination because that might delay the initiation of life-saving treatment, with potentially catastrophic consequences. The primary survey should be frequently repeated in order to promptly identify any change in the patient's physiological status. This ensures that interventions can then be introduced in a timely fashion with the objective of preventing further deteriorations.

**Table 13.1** Outline of assessments and actions included in the primary survey ABCDEF

| Assessment | Information sought | Possible resultant actions |
|---|---|---|
| **A**irway – patency | • Look for any signs of obstruction (seesaw breathing, severe recession, stridor, grunting or absent breath sounds)<br>• Note if conscious level diminished patient may not maintain airway patency<br>　• Endotracheal tube size/length, patency and if secure (if already intubated) | • Give oxygen<br>• Reposition head<br>• Apply jaw thrust<br>• Suction if indicated<br>• Insert oropharyngeal or nasopharyngeal airway<br>• Insert laryngeal mask airway<br>• Intubate if other manoeuvres fail<br>• Reassess |
| **B**reathing – adequacy | • Look for potentially life-threatening conditions<br>• Is the patient breathing?<br>• Look, listen and feel for signs of respiratory distress<br>• Look for cyanosis/pallor<br>• Measure the respiratory rate<br>• Are the breath sounds equal?<br>• Intercostal/subcostal/sternal recession and suprasternal retraction present?<br>• Head bob, nasal flare<br>• Measure the oxygen saturations<br>• Note any periods of apnoea<br>• Inspired oxygen requirement – trend<br>• Blood gas results<br>• Transilluminate the chest for a pneumothorax (infants and young children) | • Administer oxygen<br>• Support breathing with bag–valve–mask or anaesthetic circuit<br>• Consider intubation<br>• Aspirate chest if pneumothorax is suspected<br>• Adjust/optimise ventilator settings if appropriate |
| **C**irculation – adequacy | • Look at colour – cyanosis pallor<br>• Listen to the heart sounds – rate and rhythm/gallop/murmurs<br>• Assess for hypovolaemia:<br>　• Are the peripheries cold?<br>　• What is the capillary refill time (CRT)?<br>　• Is the heart rate elevated?<br>• Assess the pulses:<br>　• Reduced in shock<br>　• In infants may be severely reduced in critically obstructed systemic circulation (aortic stenosis) or even absent (coarctation of the aorta)<br>• Measure the blood pressure<br>• Assess CRT<br>• Assess liver size<br>• Are there any signs of haemorrhage, e.g. from trachea, oesophagus, rectum, umbilicus or other traumatic injury? | • Obtain vascular access:<br>　• IV cannula<br>　• Umbilical venous catheter<br>　• Intraosseous needle<br>• Control visible bleeding<br>　• Blood samples for blood gas, blood glucose, full blood count, urea and electrolytes and blood culture<br>　• Consider a fluid bolus 10-20 ml/kg of a balanced crystalloid<br>　• Consider ordering blood products – transfuse if haemoglobin is low<br>　• Intra-arterial access<br>　• Consider inotropes<br>　• Give antibiotics<br>　• Consider prostaglandin infusion in infants with suspected congenital heart disease<br>　• Reassess |

**Table 13.1**  (Continued)

| Assessment | Information sought | Possible resultant actions |
|---|---|---|
| | • Are there signs of an acute abdomen, pelvic fracture or scalp swelling (in neonates suggestive of sub-aponeurotic haemorrhage)? | |
| **D**isability/dextrose | • Assess level of consciousness:<br>  • AVPU<br>  • Glasgow Coma Scale<br>• Check blood glucose<br>• Examine pupil size and reactivity<br>• Feel anterior fontanelle<br>• Assess posture and tone<br>• Lateralising signs | • Reconsider ABC if conscious level is reduced – is airway safe?<br>• Give dextrose bolus if indicated by low blood sugar<br>• Maintain $pCO_2$ in normal range |
| **E**xposure | • Measure core temperature<br>• Undress patient completely and examine top to toe, front to back (prevent excessive cooling during this process)<br>• Look for rashes, wounds and lesions | • Consider warming or cooling |
| **F**amily | • Enquire of any immediate relevant history, e.g. diabetes, epilepsy | |

During the primary survey continuous monitoring of the following vital signs should be started (if not already undertaken):

- Peripheral oxygen saturation ($SpO_2$)
- Heart rate (via electrocardiogram (ECG) or pulse oximetry)
- Blood pressure (non-invasive initially; invasive as indicated)
- Capillary refill
- ECG
- Temperature (core and peripheral)

## Monitoring during the primary survey

The aim of the primary survey is to identify and treat any potentially life-threatening conditions. This assessment process takes into account the history of events leading up to the referral and a physical examination and is followed by appropriate, goal directed, treatment. During this phase arrangements should be made to establish continuous monitoring of the patient in order to ascertain the patient's baseline observations and to track changes in their condition (Box 13.2). The effectiveness of resuscitation is indicated by an improvement in the patient's clinical status. It is therefore important that this is measured and recorded frequently. If the patient's condition deteriorates at any stage the ABC assessment must be repeated, starting with A.

## Box 13.2  Monitoring vital signs starts during the primary survey

- Respiratory rate
- Peripheral oxygen saturation
- Heart rate
- Blood pressure
- Pulse pressure
- Capillary refill time
- Chest leads (ECG rhythm and waveform)
- Temperature (core and peripheral)
- Urinary output
- AVPU or Glasgow Coma Scale

## 13.3 Secondary survey (reassessment and planning definitive care)

Once any potentially life-threatening conditions have been either treated or excluded, a comprehensive history can be taken and a thorough examination carried out to plan definitive care. During this phase the treatment already initiated should continue as necessary. Regular reassessments should continue throughout this phase.

The objective of the reassessment ABCDEF is to refine the diagnosis and treatment through the identification of new signs and symptoms. These will either support, or refute, the working diagnosis. The plans for ongoing investigation and treatment can then be refined. These will include decisions about the best location to continue delivering the patient's care.

The key components of the secondary survey are:

- A detailed medical history
- A full physical examination
- Clinical investigations
- Formulation of a definitive plan for continuing care

Once again this is best structured using the ABCDEF approach.

Patients should be resuscitated and stable before moving between centres or even between units within the receiving hospital wherever possible. This may not always be achievable when they require care modalities that are not available in the referring unit. Such exceptions might be for advanced cardiorespiratory support such as high frequency ventilation or extracorporeal membrane oxygenation, or for time critical interventions such as neurosurgery. In all cases an ongoing need for active resuscitation and stabilisation during transfer should be the exception not the rule. A systematic approach to rapid clinical assessment, for use both prior to departure and during transfer, is extremely useful.

## 13.4 Summary

When becoming involved with the care of a patient for potential transfer it is important to follow exactly the same rules that are applied as the initial responder to an emergency. This is delivered through the use of the ABCDEF structure using a primary survey to seek out and treat any potentially life-threatening problems followed by secondary survey ABCDEF reassessment and planning of definitive care. The assessment regarding appropriateness and need for transfer form part of the reassessment phase.

# CHAPTER 14
# Clinical considerations for neonates and children

---

## Learning outcomes

After reading this chapter, you will be able to:
- Outline a structured clinical approach to the assessment and initial care of transfer patients, with specific reference to the key considerations for neonates and children
- Identify important physiological differences between infants and small children and adults
- Discuss the specific conditions that may need to be considered in the paediatric and neonatal population

---

## 14.1 Introduction

The previous sections of this book have described the general principles of ACCEPT which can be applied to any transfer situation. The following chapter may be used as a reminder of the key principles involved in the assessment and initial stabilisation of infants and children prior to transfer. It also includes advice regarding the differences between infants and small children and adults and the management of specific conditions in children and infants as they relate to transport.

The primary survey (for infants called the initial approach assessment and stabilisation of any potentially life-threatening problems) followed by secondary survey (for infants called the reassessment and planning of definitive care) will be outlined in this chapter.

## 14.2 Clinical assessment

The ABCDEF approach to a primary survey is described in Chapter 13 with reference to all age groups. In this chapter further detailed considerations will be discussed that are pertinent primarily to neonatal and paediatric patients (Box 14.1)

---

### Box 14.1 ABCDEF approach

**A**   Airway assessment and control
**B**   Breathing
**C**   Circulation
**D**   Disability and Dextrose
**E**   Exposure (including temperature in neonates and children) and Everything else
**F**   Family

---

Before describing in more detail the ABCDEF approach to primary survey some key physiological differences between infants and small children and adults will be briefly reviewed.

---

*Neonatal, Adult and Paediatric Safe Transfer and Retrieval: A Practical Approach to Transfers*, First Edition.
Edited by Bernard Foëx, Peter-Marc Fortune and Cassie Lawn.
© 2019 John Wiley & Sons Ltd. Published 2019 by John Wiley & Sons Ltd.

## 14.3 Physiological and anatomical considerations in infants and children

### Airway and breathing

Respiratory decompensation in children can be rapid, especially in infants. This is because of the anatomical and physiological features that are unique to this group. These features may be particularly pronounced in newborn and preterm infants, and are listed in Table 14.1. Emboldened features may make intubation more difficult.

**Table 14.1** Anatomical differences between infants and larger children

| Anatomy | Effect on airway/breathing |
|---|---|
| **Large occiput** | ↑ Neck flexion potentially causing airway obstruction |
| **Large tongue** | ↑ Risk of airway obstruction |
| **Floppy epiglottis** | ↑ Risk of airway obstruction |
| **Larynx anterior/cephalad** | ↑ Risk of difficult intubation |
| Short trachea | ↑ Risk of bronchial intubation |
| **Trachea angled posteriorly** | ↑ Risk of difficult intubation |
| Low pharyngeal muscle tone | ↑ Risk of airway obstruction |
| Small nares | ↑ Airway resistance (<3 months usually nasal breathers) |
| Cricoid cartilage | Narrowest point up to 8 years |
| Narrow airways | ↑ Airway resistance |
| Compliant airways | May collapse with increased respiratory effort |
| Compliant chest wall | Inefficient delivery of respiratory muscle effort |
| Barrel shaped chest | Horizontal ribs reduce the contribution of chest wall movement to lung inflation |
| Flattened diaphragm | Reduced diaphragmatic movement |
| Immature respiratory muscles | Reduced effectiveness of forced expiration, e.g. cough |

Oxygen consumption in the newborn is approximately 7 ml/kg/min (around twice that of adults).

Gas available for exchange at the alveolar level (alveolar minute ventilation) is determined by the tidal volume, respiratory rate and dead space.

Infants have a relative inability to increase their tidal volumes. This is because they have a compliant rib cage, the effect of which may be exacerbated by stiff lungs (e.g. in surfactant deficiency). **Therefore, respiratory distress may often serve as an early sign of illness in an infant.** For example, tachypnoea may develop to increase minute ventilation in response to a metabolic acidosis with or without raised carbon dioxide levels.

As dead space is usually constant, inadequate gas for exchange at the alveolar level may arise from a reduction in tidal volumes or respiratory rate. This may occur either due to pulmonary pathology or reduced effort as the child tires.

Newborns also have a relatively low functional residual capacity (FRC). This is the volume of gas left in the lungs at the end of normal tidal expiration. This gas acts as a reservoir for oxygen and prevents alveolar collapse. The reduction in FRC may be further exacerbated in respiratory diseases such as hyaline membrane disease or pneumonia. Grunting (forced expirations against a partially closed glottis) increases FRC and helps recruit alveoli.

Intercostal, subcostal, supraclavicular and sternal retraction result from increased muscle effort, to maintain adequate ventilation, in the presence of a compliant chest wall. Nasal flaring signals a child's effort to maximise air entry through the nose by minimising upper airway resistance.

### Circulation

Shock is a result of failure to supply tissues with adequate oxygen and remove waste products of metabolism. Adequate oxygen delivery to the tissues requires a sufficient cardiac output *and* a sufficient blood oxygen content. Cardiac output (CO) is the amount of blood pumped into the circulation. It is dependent on both heart rate and stroke volume:

$$CO = \text{heart rate (HR)} \times \text{stroke volume (SV)}$$

The stroke volume is determined by how well the ventricle fills during diastole and its ability to pump blood forward during systole.

The newborn myocardium is less compliant than that of the older child, therefore infants are less able than adults to vary their stroke volume (Table 14.2). They are consequently more dependent on increasing their heart rate to increase their cardiac output. This is especially so in the preterm infant. **Tachycardia is often the first sign of cardiovascular compromise in infants.**

**Table 14.2** Normal heart rates

| Age | Heart rate Beats per minute 5th–95th centile |
|---|---|
| Birth | 120–170 |
| 1 month | |
| 3 months | 115–160 |
| 6 months | 110–160 |
| 12 months | |
| 18 months | 100–155 |
| 2 years | 100–150 |
| 3 years | 90–140 |
| 4 years | 80–135 |
| 5 years | |
| 6 years | 80–130 |
| 7 years | |
| 8 years | 70–120 |
| 9 years | |
| 10 years | |
| 11 years | |
| 12 years | 65–115 |
| 14 years | 60–110 |

Anaemia causes a more rapid onset of shock as there is a reduced oxygen carrying capacity in the blood. Conversely, significant polycythaemia makes the blood more viscous. This may inhibit flow through small vessels, consequently reducing tissue perfusion and worsening pre-existing pulmonary hypertension.

The factors affecting stroke volume are preload, afterload and myocardial contractility. Preload refers to the volume of blood that flows into the heart during diastole. A reduction in preload reduces stroke volume. This may commonly occur secondary to hypovolaemia, causing reduced venous return and filling. Hypovolaemia may be due to:

- High fluid loss or 'third spacing' – e.g. with necrotising enterocolitis
- Sepsis – causing capillary leak and poor vascular tone
- Anaphylaxis – poor vascular tone (functional hypovolaemia)

Raised intrathoracic pressures may also reduce venous return, e.g. with a tension pneumothorax or secondary to high positive pressure ventilation. In rare circumstances a cardiac tamponade may directly reduce filling of the heart. Severe tachycardias may also result in such short periods of diastole that the heart is unable to fill adequately in the time available.

Contractility is a measure of the shortening ability of the cardiac muscle fibres. This describes the effectiveness of the pumping ability of the heart. Poor contractility reduces cardiac output and is associated with:

- Hypoxia
- Hypoglycaemia
- Sepsis (e.g. group B streptococcal infection)
- Some types of congenital heart disease
- Hydrops fetalis
- Myocarditis
- Hypocalcaemia
- Abnormal cardiac conduction

Afterload is the pressure the ventricles must pump against to eject blood. Constricted arterial blood vessels in both the peripheral and pulmonary circulations increase afterload and reduce cardiac output. Increased afterload in obstructive congenital cardiac lesions such as aortic stenosis or coarctation of the aorta can lead to reduced cardiac output and may rapidly lead to severe cardiac failure.

### Blood pressure

Blood pressure (Tables 14.3 and 14.4) is often used as a surrogate measure for adequate cardiac output. In illness, dysregulation of blood supply to vital organs may not enable adequate perfusion in the face of a normal blood pressure. However, in most situations maintaining an adequate blood pressure will usually ensure that the vital organs are adequately perfused. Further evidence may be secured by monitoring the child's urine output. In the absence of renal disease or high blood osmolality (e.g. diabetic ketoacidosis), a urine output of 1–2 ml/kg/h suggests that the kidneys are adequately perfused. This can be particularly useful when blood pressure is borderline. Acid–base balance may also be monitored in this regard, as low output states will usually be reflected by a metabolic acidosis.

**Table 14.3** Systolic blood pressure (BP) by age

| Age | BP systolic | | |
| --- | --- | --- | --- |
| | 5th centile | 50th centile | 95th centile |
| Birth | 65–75 | 80–90 | 105 |
| 1 month | | | |
| 3 months | | | |
| 6 months | | | |
| 12 months | 70–75 | 85–95 | |
| 18 months | | | |
| 2 years | 70–80 | 85–100 | 110 |
| 3 years | | | |
| 4 years | | | |
| 5 years | 80–90 | 90–110 | 111–120 |
| 6 years | | | |
| 7 years | | | |
| 8 years | | | |
| 9 years | | | |
| 10 years | | | |
| 11 years | | | |
| 12 years | 90–105 | 100–120 | 125–140 |
| 14 years | | | |
| Adult | | | |

**Table 14.4** Normal values on day 1 in healthy, preterm infants

| Gestation (weeks) | Systolic range (mmHg) | Diastolic range (mmHg) | Heart rate (min–max) | Mean blood pressure |
|---|---|---|---|---|
| <24 | 48–63 | 24–39 | 120–190 | 24 |
| 24–28 | 48–58 | 22–36 | 120–190 | 24–28 |
| 29–32 | 47–59 | 27–34 | 120–170 | 30 |
| >32 | 48–60 | 24–34 | 120–170 | 30 |

### Septic shock

Children with sepsis are often able to maintain their blood pressure through increased peripheral tone leading to cool extremities. This state of compensated shock masks inadequate cardiac output and may be overlooked by inexperienced clinicians. By contrast some children, particularly preterm infants, may present with reduced peripheral vascular tone; this is known as warm shock.

As sepsis progresses, children who were initially peripherally shut-down may lose homeostatic vascular control. Generalised vasodilatation results in plasma leakage (third space loss) and reduced venous return. This in turn reduces preload and therefore cardiac output. This will manifest as metabolic acidosis and ultimately hypotension. In addition, some pathogens produce toxins that directly depress cardiac contractility, further compromising cardiac output.

### Blood pressure and the brain

In healthy adults and children cerebral blood flow is controlled by autoregulation. This means that cerebral blood flow is maintained within normal limits even in the face of systemic hyper- or hypotension. This control system operates less well in ill infants, especially those who are preterm. Rapid fluctuations in blood pressure (notably in the presence of hypoxia or acidosis) increase the risk of altered cerebral perfusion causing hypoxic injury or intraventricular haemorrhage, particularly in preterms.

### Circulatory changes at birth

In utero blood is oxygenated via the placenta. The foramen ovale and ductus arteriosus are patent, and the lungs have a high vascular resistance and there is very little pulmonary blood flow. Blood bypasses the lungs by flowing straight from the right to left atrium via the foramen ovale, or by flowing from the pulmonary artery into the aorta via the ductus arteriosus.

At birth the lungs are aerated and the pulmonary vascular resistance falls and blood starts to flow through the lungs. Blood leaves the lungs and fills the left atrium and flow via the foramen ovale gradually reduces as left atrial pressure rises and usually ceases physiologically within a few hours of birth. The ductus arteriosus contracts in response to increased oxygen levels in the blood. The pressure in the pulmonary artery also decreases and flow through the duct diminishes. The duct is usually functionally closed within the first day of life.

Failure to aerate the lungs at birth and to establish adequate blood flow through them results in hypoxia. If this is prolonged then the pulmonary circulation maintains a high resistance that manifests as persistent pulmonary hypertension which encourages flow through these fetal structures. Congenital structural abnormalities can also disrupt the progress of normal cardiovascular adaptation at birth. Understanding fetal and newborn cardiovascular physiology is key to recognising the significance of clinical findings in the sick infant.

## 14.4  Primary survey

Table 14.5 outlines the primary survey of an infant or child using ABCDEF. Any life-threatening problems should be treated as they are identified, and this primary survey will be followed by a secondary survey. During the transport process it will not always be possible to undertake all necessary investigations, but a provisional diagnosis and appropriate investigations are an integral part of planning a transport to the correct place at the correct time and are therefore integral to the transport process

**Table 14.5** Outline of assessments and actions in initial ABCDEF

| Assessment | Information sought | Possible resultant actions |
|---|---|---|
| **A**irway – patency | • Look for any signs of obstruction (seesaw breathing, severe recession, no breath sounds in complete obstruction)<br>• Note if conscious level is diminished, infant or child may not maintain airway patency | • Reposition head<br>• Apply jaw thrust<br>• Suction if indicated<br>• Insert oropharyngeal airway<br>• Insert laryngeal mask airway<br>• Intubate if other manoeuvres fail<br>• Give oxygen<br>• Reassess |
| **B**reathing – adequacy | • Look for immediately potentially life-threatening conditions<br>• Is the infant/child breathing?<br>• Look, listen and feel for signs of respiratory distress<br>• Look for cyanosis/pallor<br>• Measure the respiratory rate<br>• Are the breath sounds equal?<br>• Intercostal/subcostal/sternal recession and suprasternal retraction<br>• Head bob, nasal flare<br>• Measure the oxygen saturations (pre- and post-ductal)<br>• Apnoeas<br>• Endotracheal tube size/patency/fixation<br>• Inspired oxygen requirement – trend<br>• Blood gas results<br>• Transilluminate the chest for a pneumothorax (check chest X-ray if available) | • Administer oxygen<br>• Support breathing with bag–valve–mask or T piece<br>• Consider intubation<br>• Aspirate chest if pneumothorax is suspected<br>• Adjust/optimise ventilator settings if appropriate |
| **C**irculation – adequacy | • Look at colour: cyanosis pallor<br>• Listen to the heart sounds – rate and rhythm/gallop/murmurs<br>• Assess for hypovolaemia:<br>  • Are the peripheries cold?<br>  • What is the capillary refill time (CRT)?<br>  • Is the child tachycardic?<br>• Assess the pulses (reduced in shock or critically obstructed systemic circulation, e.g. aortic stenosis, reduced femoral pulses in coarctation of the aorta)<br>• Measure the blood pressure<br>• Assess CRT<br>• Liver size<br>• Are there any signs of haemorrhage, e.g. from umbilicus?<br>• Subaponeurotic haemorrhage? | • Obtain access:<br>  • IV cannula<br>  • Umbilical venous catheter<br>  • Intraosseous needle<br>• Control visible bleeding<br>• Blood samples for blood gas, blood sugar, full blood count, urea and electrolytes and blood culture<br>• Consider a fluid bolus 10–20 ml/kg of normal saline<br>• Consider ordering blood products – transfuse if haemoglobin is low<br>• Intra-arterial access<br>• Consider inotropes<br>• Give antibiotics<br>• Consider prostaglandin infusion<br>• Reassess |
| **D**isability/dextrose | • Assess level of consciousness:<br>  • Alert<br>  • Responsive to stimuli<br>  • Unresponsive to all stimuli<br>• Check blood glucose<br>• Examine pupil size<br>• Feel anterior fontanlle and feel the scalp – is there massive swelling crossing the suture lines suggestive of subaponeurotic bleeding?<br>• Posture and tone | • Give 2.5 ml/kg 10% dextrose if indicated<br>• Reconsider ABC in infant in light of conscious level<br>• Maintain $pCO_2$ in normal range |

**Table 14.5** (Continued)

| Assessment | Information sought | Possible resultant actions |
|---|---|---|
| **E**xposure | • Measure core temperature<br>• Undress infant/child completely and examine top to toe and front to back<br>• Look for rashes/wounds lesions | • Consider warming or cooling<br>• Reassess |
| **F**amily | • Identify any immediate relevant history | |

During primary survey monitoring the following vital signs should be started (if not already undertaken):

- Peripheral oxygen saturation ($SpO_2$)
- Heart rate
- Blood pressure
- Pulse pressure
- Capillary refill time
- Electrocardiogram (ECG)
- Temperature (core and peripheral)

Once any immediate potentially life-threatening conditions have been either treated or excluded, a comprehensive history can be taken and a thorough examination carried out. During this second phase, emergency treatment should continue as necessary. During the secondary survey the aim is to find new features and corroborative evidence to support, or refute, the working diagnosis. With this information it should then be possible to formulate plans for ongoing investigation and treatment; this will include decisions about the best location to continue this care. The key components of secondary survey are:

- A detailed medical history
- A full examination
- Appropriate investigations
- Formulation of a definitive plan for continuing care

Wherever possible, children who are in transit between referring and receiving centres should be fully resuscitated and stable before departure. This may not be possible when they require care modalities not available in the referring unit. However, the need for active resuscitation and stabilisation during transfer should be the exception not the rule. A systematic approach to rapid clinical assessment, for use both prior to departure and during transfer, promotes continual safe practice.

**Reassessment in the secondary survey should be along ABCDEF lines, but it is going to be very much guided by key clinical problem or diagnosis. Specific details of how to manage specific conditions are outlined below.**

## 14.5 Secondary survey (reassessment and planning of definitive care)

A thorough head to toe, front to back examination of the child should be carried out after the primary survey. This should be followed by additional appropriate investigations and the formulation of a definitive plan for continuing care.

Throughout the entire process it is vital that the child is continually monitored to assess the effect of treatment and to detect any worsening of their condition. If any deterioration is noted then a re-evaluation of ABCDEF is mandatory. By the end of the secondary survey a working diagnosis should be available together with a list of additional investigations and appropriate treatments. At this point plans for definitive care should determine the most appropriate place for the child.

## 14.6 Specific clinical conditions

In this section we will provide an overview of clinical considerations of a number of important paediatric and neonatal conditions that may present and require transfer (Box 14.2). This is not intended to provide an exhaustive overview; rather it presents a subset of conditions that are included because of their high incidence or because they require specialist management, that may occasionally seem counterintuitive, in order to achieve the best outcome.

## Box 14.2 Need for transfer

- Specialist treatment
- Specialist investigations
- More appropriate location for the delivery of level 0, 1, 2 or 3 care – local, specialist or supraregional

In all cases a primary survey and more detailed reassessment (detailed secondary survey) should be undertaken. The information below is provided as a supplement and consequently assumes that the structure described above is already being appropriately followed.

### Pneumothorax

A high index of suspicion regarding the possibility of a pneumothorax should be maintained in children with respiratory compromise, especially following sudden deterioration. Infants with hyaline membrane disease or children requiring high ventilator pressures are at particular risk.

Children who have developed a tension pneumothorax will become progressively more difficult to ventilate as the intrapleural pressure increases. They may rapidly develop shock, as their cardiac output falls secondary to obstruction to venous return. Diagnosis of a tension pneumothorax must be made on clinical grounds as a child can arrest in the time it takes to expose and process a chest radiograph.

If a tension pneumothorax has been diagnosed a 21 or 23 gauge butterfly or cannula attached to a three-way tap should be inserted into the second intercostal space in the mid-clavicular line. The air may then escape via the tap. This procedure provides temporary chest drainage, and a definitive chest drain must be sited as a matter of urgency.

Note, if no pneumothorax was present the passage of the needle may cause a pneumothorax. An urgent chest radiograph must always be performed in these circumstances.

### Bronchiolitis

This is a common seasonal illness that presents primarily during the winter months. Severely affected children often need to be cared for in a high dependency unit (HDU) or paediatric intensive care unit (PICU). The majority of cases are caused by respiratory syncitial virus, the remainder by other common respiratory viruses. The underlying pathophysiology is of bronchiolar obstruction secondary to inflammatory debris and oedema. Areas of atelectasis form, and ball-valve type obstruction may lead to areas of hyperinflation.

Requirement for transfer to a PICU for invasive ventilation is the result of either progressive respiratory failure or because of recurrent apnoeas. The latter may be the presenting feature of the illness in young infants, sometimes occurring before there is any obvious sign of respiratory distress. The need for ventilation can sometimes be avoided by using non-invasive support techniques such as high flow nasal cannula (HFNC) humidified oxygen or continuous positive airway pressure (CPAP) to reduce the work of breathing and to prevent atelectasis. This may be delivered in HDUs in some centres but in others will require transfer to a PICU. The children who are most likely to require intubation and ventilation are those with a history of chronic lung disease of prematurity (CLDP), newborn infants or infants with an underlying cardiorespiratory abnormality.

Once ventilated, oxygen saturations of 88–92% and permissive hypercapnia (keeping the pH >7.2) are acceptable. Using positive end expiratory pressure (PEEP) in the range 6–15 cmH$_2$O should be employed to improve oxygenation and ventilation/perfusion (VQ) mismatch by minimising atelectasis. A target of 5–7 ml/kg of tidal volume is useful to guide in establishing the most appropriate peak inspiratory pressure (PIP), and a respiratory rate of 30 with an inspiratory time of 0.8 seconds is a reasonable starting point for ventilation. During transfer, endotracheal tube (ET) obstruction by secretions should be anticipated.

Transferring staff must ensure that there is a plentiful supply of appropriate gauge suction catheters, and portable suction must be available at all times. The best way to manage these children on the PICU is to allow spontaneous synchronised ventilation; however, during transfer they will often be paralysed to prevent excessive movement and coughing which may displace the ET tube.

A common issue encountered in these infants is whether to transfer using CPAP/HFNC or to escalate to invasive ventilation. The best place to deliver care will be determined by local circumstances. Non-invasive ventilation can be performed on general paediatric wards where provision has been made to allow high dependency care. The risk of transferring a child with CPAP/HFNC is that they become unstable en route and require intubation and ventilation as an emergency procedure. Having to undertake this process in the back of an ambulance is best avoided! When a child is commenced on CPAP in a referring centre with the resources to provide appropriate HDU care it is appropriate to wait and see if they stabilise. Any significant deterioration should generate a prompt clinical review followed by intubation, ventilation and transfer where required. Transfer on CPAP/HFNC under the direction of a consultant may be appropriate.

## Epiglottitis

Although this has become much less common since the introduction of the *Haemophilus influenzae* type B (HiB) vaccination it does still occur. Epiglottitis can be caused by other organisms. It has become more common in recent years secondary to HiB vaccine failures.

The child will typically present with a very short history of fever, drooling and stridor. They appear flushed and hot. Upset to the child must be minimised. Painful or potentially upsetting examinations or procedures are absolutely contraindicated. Senior help must always be promptly summoned. If there are signs of upper airway obstruction, the child should be intubated by a consultant intensivist or anaesthetist utilising a technique of gaseous induction. It is recommended that an ENT surgeon is also present and ready to perform an emergency tracheostomy if necessary. Where possible, a nasotracheal tube should be placed to optimise later management on the PICU. This will usually be achieved as a secondary procedure once the operator has secured the airway via an oral ET tube. Elective reintubation should not be undertaken if there is any doubt of success.

The challenges for this condition lie with the initial induction and intubation, and less with the transport – except to say that security of the ET tube is of paramount importance. The child should be sedated and paralysed for the transfer and the ET tube fixed with tape firmly to the face, ensuring that it does not move. End-tidal $CO_2$ monitoring is mandatory to facilitate immediate recognition of a displaced or blocked tube. If accidental extubation were to occur, then a gum elastic bougie should be available to assist in correct replacement. If it is not possible either to reintubate or to bag–valve–mask ventilate, a laryngeal mask may allow some ventilation to be achieved, although in the context of a severe epiglottitis it may be that the only way to oxygenate will be to perform a needle cricothyroidotomy.

In practice, with an experienced retrieval team, the incidence of accidental extubation is extremely low. The likeliest points for it to occur are when moving the child between the bed and stretcher, and on loading and unloading the stretcher in the ambulance. At these times, one team member should be allocated the specific role of ensuring that all ventilator tubing and monitoring cables are in a secure position and are not likely to snag. It is advisable to disconnect the ventilator from the tube for the short time it takes to move the child from the bed to trolley.

These children are septic, therefore in addition to airway management remember that they may require cardiovascular support. This may include fluid boluses and inotrope infusions. Consideration should be given to placing a central line prior to transfer.

## Upper airway disease

Croup is the most common upper airway emergency requiring intubation and ventilation. Fortunately, this is needed in only a small fraction of cases. The child will typically present with coryzal symptoms, low grade fever, harsh barking cough and stridor.

The key indication for intubation is worsening respiratory distress. This may manifest as severe sternal and intercostal recession plus or minus hypoxia. Eventually, even in a moderately severe case, the child may become exhausted and require intubation to maintain adequate ventilation. Airway obstruction is always worst when the child is upset and consequently trying to generate high gas flows through their obstructed upper airway. Temporary relief may be achieved through the use of nebulised adrenaline (0.4 ml/kg of 1:1000 adrenaline up to maximum of 5 ml). Many children with croup will be free of stridor for a period after this treatment. Some will then develop worsening stridor after an initial response to adrenaline. This probably happens not because of rebound hyperaemia of their upper airway mucosa, but because of severe underlying inflammation. The need for an adrenaline nebuliser should always prompt an immediate consultant review. The need for multiple adrenaline nebulisers almost invariably indicates the requirement for prompt intubation and ventilation.

With croup, as with all causes of upper airway obstruction, a requirement for supplementary oxygen in order to maintain normal saturations is worrying. All such children should be reviewed by a consultant immediately.

The glottic swelling often means that only a relatively narrow tube can be passed; standard tubes are often too short for the child. Special 'croup tubes' are available which are longer than standard, narrow diameter tubes.

The need for tube security applies here as it does in epiglottitis and all other upper airway obstruction.

## Acute on chronic respiratory failure

Many admissions to PICUs result from respiratory infections in children who have pre-existing lung disease, most commonly CLDP. This will usually be evident from the history given by the parents, although there may be additional clues from the appearance of the chest X-ray (CXR), and the presence of a partially compensated respiratory acidosis.

Children with chronic lung disease often have coexistent areas of hyperinflation and collapse. The CXRs may be difficult to interpret. Careful inspection for a pneumothorax is important prior to departure. Consideration should be given to draining even a small pneumothorax in these circumstances. The CXR should be used in conjunction with oxygen saturations and blood gas analysis to select appropriate ventilator settings. These infants often respond well to a moderately high PEEP and relatively long inspiratory times; this will maintain a high mean airway pressure whilst allowing peak pressures to be kept to a minimum. As with patients with bronchiolitis, aiming for oxygen saturations of 88–92% and a strategy of permissive hypercapnia is a reasonable approach. Careful attention to appropriate sedation is especially important in children with chronic lung disease as they may have secondary pulmonary hypertension.

Many of these children will require a long period of stabilisation prior to transport. There is often a degree of experimentation needed with ventilator settings – there is no general 'ventilator recipe' that will suit all.

## Severe pneumonia

It is relatively unusual for a bacterial or viral pneumonia to cause respiratory failure severe enough to require ventilation in a previously well child beyond early infancy. Such a requirement should prompt enquiry into evidence of a pre-existing respiratory, neurological or immunological problem.

With a severe bacterial pneumonia, marked respiratory deterioration may be caused by an empyema. An ultrasound scan of the chest will allow evaluation of the presence and location of any pleural fluid. The insertion of a chest drain to relieve even a small collection may produce a rapid, significant improvement.

Children with a bacterial pneumonia may have significant systemic sepsis, so their haemodynamic status must be evaluated carefully (heart rate, perfusion, urine output, lactate). Appropriate volume resuscitation should be administered and consideration given to the insertion of a central venous line and inotrope infusion.

## Acute respiratory distress syndrome

Acute respiratory distress syndrome (ARDS) is the term used to describe severe respiratory failure associated with bilateral pulmonary infiltrates on CXR without evidence of cardiogenic pulmonary oedema. It may result from extrapulmonary or pulmonary causes.

- Pulmonary:
  - Pneumonia
  - Aspiration of gastric contents
  - Smoke inhalation
  - Near drowning
- Extrapulmonary:
  - Sepsis
  - Trauma
  - Burns

This list of causes is far from exhaustive, but covers the commonest seen in children.

The pathophysiology is of a severe inflammatory oedema caused by vascular endothelial injury and increased capillary permeability. VQ mismatch causes severe hypoxia, and areas of consolidation develop in a dependent fashion, causing a heterogeneous decrease in pulmonary compliance. In extrapulmonary ARDS the treatment will be complicated by the predisposing cause, and the mortality of the condition is related to this rather than the presence of ARDS per se. The prognosis for pulmonary ARDS in a previously well child is very good if treated in a PICU.

## Congenital heart disease

Advances in paediatric cardiac surgery and in postoperative care of children with congenital heart disease (CHD) has led some to argue that the time of greatest danger for these children is not perioperatively, but during the time period before they reach the specialist centre. Early discharge of babies who appear initially well means that many of these babies may present in extremis to emergency departments. One in four of babies dying in the first week of life from cardiac disease did not have their diagnosis recognised prior to presentation in extremis.

A provisional diagnosis may be available locally but this is rarely made by a paediatric cardiologist. Therefore, management decisions may not be clear-cut and should be discussed with a paediatric intensivist or cardiologist.

The detail of the underlying anatomy is unimportant in the initial stages of resuscitation and management. The principles of ABCDEF are just the same as in other settings, with the qualification that normal oxygen saturations may not be achievable (or desirable). The key feature in addition to the standard resuscitation process is that of considering ductal patency. CHD presents acutely in one of three ways:

- Cyanosis, but otherwise looking well (alert, active, minimal or no tachypnoea)
- Cyanosis and sick (respiratory distress)
- Shock (often indistinguishable from sepsis)

In nearly all cases, maintaining the patency of the ductus arteriosus that connects the systemic and pulmonary circulations is paramount. It is often the physiological closing of the ductus that precipitates clinical deterioration and presentation. Measures to reopen a closing ductus may therefore produce a rapid improvement in the child's condition.

Ductal patency may be maintained by prostaglandin E1 (alprostadil) or prostaglandin E2 (dinoprostone) (consult the BNFC for dose ranges). The key side effects of these agents are apnoea and hypotension. These both occur with increasing frequency as the dose increases. If apnoeas occur, intubation and ventilation should be performed, and hypotension should be treated by volume resuscitation and inotropes. The infusion of prostaglandin must *not* be discontinued.

Note that the names of the alternative prostaglandins are very similar and may also be confused with other agents used in the neonatal period. Consequently, extra vigilance is advised when prescribing and administering these agents.

### Cyanosed and well

An example of this category is transposition of the great arteries.

The infant who is cyanosed and well can be managed with a prostaglandin infusion, and observed for apnoeas, but does not necessarily need to be electively intubated. If they are stable for several hours on low or standard doses of prostaglandin, they can be transferred without intubation – apnoeas usually occur early after institution of high dose prostaglandin.

### Respiratory distress and cyanosis

Examples include pulmonary atresia, severe tetralogy of Fallot and non-cardiac examples, e.g. persistent pulmonary hypertension of the newborn.

Infants with respiratory distress and cyanosis may have a pulmonary rather than a cardiac problem. A nitrogen wash-out test (breathing 100% oxygen for 10 minutes) that shows a rise in saturations and a $PaO_2 > 15$ kPa, makes a respiratory cause more likely. However, a failure to improve oxygenation may simply reflect an intrapulmonary shunt, or cardiac shunting secondary to pulmonary hypertension. It does not confirm cardiac disease. It is reasonable to start a prostaglandin infusion, intubate and ventilate the child for respiratory failure, and transfer to a specialist centre for a definitive diagnosis.

### Shocked Infants

Infants who present with shock may have sepsis or a duct-dependent circulation secondary to systemic outflow obstruction (e.g. hypoplastic left heart syndrome, critical aortic stenosis, coarctation of the aorta). The hallmark signs are poor systemic perfusion, metabolic acidosis and weak or impalpable pulses. It is usually reasonable to start a prostaglandin infusion and to treat for sepsis with broad-spectrum antibiotics. There will often be a good response to prostaglandin in those with CHD and those with sepsis will often show some response to fluid boluses. However, distinguishing the two is only really possible with echocardiography.

Key indications for considering prostaglandins are:

- Cyanosis with no respiratory cause
- Cyanosis with a murmur
- Abnormal (absent) pulses

The more unwell an infant is, the lower the threshold should be for starting prostaglandins.

Once improvement is achieved by reopening the duct, the focus should shift to balancing the systemic and pulmonary circulations. In hypoplastic left heart syndrome, two parallel circuits are in operation. Blood in the right ventricle can be pumped into the lungs via the pulmonary artery, or into the aorta via the ductus. Ideally this should be in a 1:1 ratio. Too much blood to the lungs will be at the expense of the systemic circulation, manifest by a continuing metabolic acidosis, poor urine output and relatively high oxygen saturations. Increasing the $FiO_2$ to try and achieve high saturations may lower pulmonary vascular resistance, and promote this systemic steal, so it is important to use a ventilator that allows low $FiO_2$ (or air) to be administered. Saturations of 70–80% are a reasonable target – bear in mind this will be the saturation target that surgeons will be aiming for in the first stage of repair, and that will sustain the child for several months or even years.

## Cardiomyopathy, myocarditis and pericarditis

Intrinsic heart disease is rare in childhood compared with adults. Cardiomyopathy and myocarditis may present as congestive cardiac failure at any age, and the clinical features overlap, making it difficult to differentiate the two at acute presentation. Other children will have had the diagnosis of cardiomyopathy established long before they present to a PICU team. In both cases the challenge is to maintain sufficient cardiac output to maintain systemic oxygen delivery. Intensive care unit management will be along the same lines until there is improvement in the underlying condition, but some may eventually require full support with extracorporeal membrane oxygenation (ECMO).

These diagnoses should be considered in any child with shock or pulmonary oedema, enlarged liver (before any fluid resuscitation) and an enlarged cardiac contour on CXR. Echocardiography and an ECG will confirm the diagnosis, and allow the estimation of cardiac function. This is quoted as fractional shortening (FS) in children (adults often have the ejection fraction reported). FS is normally in the range of 28–42%. It is a two-dimensional measure of how much the left ventricle contracts during systole as a fraction of its original dimensions.

Intubation and ventilation may be beneficial in children with a very low FS. This is achieved by reducing left ventricular afterload and also the work of breathing, which may be significant because of their pulmonary oedema. However, these benefits may be outweighed by the risk of induction and intubation; the vasodilatory and negative inotropic effects of the anaesthetic agents can cause cardiac arrest. Induction agents tend to be chosen to minimise these effects. Fentanyl and ketamine tend to be popular in this situation. Resuscitation drugs should be drawn up in readiness, and the child transferred to the safest environment available.

Once ventilated, the need for inotropes should be evaluated and they should be started if appropriate. The choice of inotrope is determined by personal preference rather than evidence, but dopamine is a reasonable starting point. Adrenaline should be considered if there is no response. Administration details can be found in the BFNC. The desired therapeutic end point is to achieve an adequate cardiac output. If available, this can be measured directly by the PiCCO or CardioQ™ systems. Otherwise, optimisation of cardiac output may be estimated through measurement of surrogate markers, such as heart rate, peripheral perfusion, arterial lactate concentration, urine output and blood pressure (continuously measured from an arterial line). Preload should be optimised judiciously using small (5 ml/kg) boluses of fluid and close monitoring of response of end points. Ventilation often requires a high PEEP if there is pulmonary oedema. In children with severe, bloody pulmonary oedema, constant suctioning of the ET tube is seldom helpful – the ventilator should be reconnected and high PEEP (10–15 cmH$_2$O) applied.

Children with pericarditis uncommonly present to intensive care; when they do it is because of a pericardial effusion causing tamponade. The most common setting for this is the cardiac intensive care unit postoperatively, but occasionally effusions present weeks later in postoperative children. Other causes are connective tissue disorders and malignant invasion of the pericardium. Like children with cardiomyopathy, induction of anaesthesia to facilitate drainage can be a high risk procedure, and unless in extremis it is probably advisable not to undertake this outside of a specialist centre. The decision about whether to intubate these children prior to transfer will be dictated by their clinical status. Unless they are in extremis, it may be safer to transfer them unintubated as soon as possible to the specialist centre.

## Dysrhythmias

Dysrhythmia requiring PICU transfer is usually due to a sustained supraventricular tachycardia (SVT) in infancy, or ventricular tachycardia (VT) in children who have been poisoned by agents such as tricyclic antidepressants or who have an underlying cardiomyopathy or myocarditis.

### *Supraventricular tachycardia*

This typically presents with a heart rate of 220–250 beats/min in infants. They usually tolerate this poorly. It generally takes a few hours for them to develop marked cardiac failure. The APLS SVT algorithm should be followed (see *Advanced Paediatric Life Support* 6e (Samuels and Wieteska, 2016), Figure 7.4).

There can be a problem differentiating SVT from sinus tachycardia in children. Sinus tachycardia secondary to hypovolaemia or sepsis will typically vary in rate in response to fluid boluses or handling, whereas the rate in SVT remains fixed. It may be helpful to fax the ECG to a paediatric cardiologist. It is important to try to capture a rhythm strip for this purpose. The administration of adenosine with continuous ECG monitoring can be a useful diagnostic tool in this scenario.

### *Ventricular tachycardia*

Ventricular tachycardia should be treated according to the APLS VT algorithm (see *Advanced Paediatric Life Support* 6e (Samuels and Wieteska, 2016), Figure 7.5).

## 14.7 Specific neonatal considerations and conditions

### Airway and breathing

In the neonatal period it is vital to appreciate the immaturity of the lungs and the fact that they are easily damaged (particularly in the extreme preterm). Ventilatory strategies are therefore aimed at minimising damage to the lungs (volutrauma and barotrauma) whilst ensuring adequate oxygenation and ventilation.

A strategy of permissive hypercapnia and relative hypoxia is employed in the preterm infant.

### Circulation

Maintenance fluids are usually given as 10% dextrose. In the first 24–48 hours it is not usually necessary to add sodium or potassium. A rate of 60–100 ml/kg/day is recommended depending on gestation. Maintenance of blood sugar is important (aim to keep above 2.6 mmol/l).

### Disabilty

Therapeutic hypothermia is a standard specialist therapy for newborn infants with hypoxic ischaemic brain injury. There is some evidence that suggests it may be neuroprotective in some asphyxiated older children if the correct regime is used. Many neonatal intensive care units now cool infants following asphyxial injury to core temperatures of 33–34 °C for 72 hours. Outside specialist centres this is not currently routine practice. In all cases close attention should be paid to the avoidance of hyperthermia as this is known to be damaging to the hypoxic brain. It is advisable to keep the core temperature at 36.5–37 °C in these circumstances. The evidence to support this practice in older children following traumatic brain injury remains inconclusive.

## Exposure

Very immature and low birth weight babies are particularly vulnerable to cold. Hypothermia increases oxygen demand and adversely affects blood clotting; low temperatures in the preterm infant are associated with a poorer outcome. Therefore minimisation of heat loss is an urgent priority in all infants and especially preterm ones. Premature and low birth weight infants have a high surface area and lose heat through the following mechanisms:

- Convection
  - From exposed skin to surrounding air
  - Exacerbated in a draught
- Radiation
  - From the surface of the baby to cooler surfaces
  - May be offset by using a radiant heater
- Evaporation
  - Heat is lost as water evaporates from the skin
  - Preterm infants are especially vulnerable
  - Minimised by the use of humidity or 'waterproofing' the infant with plastic sheet or bubble wrap
- Conduction
  - Though contact with cooler surfaces
  - Reduced by using warm bedclothes and maintaining that temperature with chemically activated gel mattress, such as a Transwarmer™

Other practical measures to reduce thermal stress that should be considered are:

- Minimise exposure time for examinations
- Use portholes if the infant is in an incubator
- Minimise draughts and warm the room/ambulance
- Nurse in warmed, humidified incubator
- Dress the infant in a hat
- Prewarm the transport incubator to 39–40 °C
- Humidify inspired gases
- Use a radiant heat source if not in an incubator
- Continually monitor temperature
- Consider delaying patient transfer until their temperature is normal

At delivery very premature infants should be placed, still wet, in a food-grade plastic bag, leaving the head out. When the infant is then placed under a radiant heat source this creates a warm, moist microenvironment for the infant which is very effective at maintaining temperature.

## Infection

The possibility of infection should always be considered in these infants. It may be difficult to differentiate between congenital pneumonia and respiratory distress syndrome on CXR. Therefore, most of these babies should be treated with antibiotics. A typical antibiotic regime would be intravenous benzyl penicillin + gentamicin or cefotaxime as a sole agent.

## Hyaline membrane disease (respiratory distress syndrome)

Surfactant deficiency is almost universal in infants born at less than 28 weeks' gestation. In many centres, non-invasive respiratory support strategies such as CPAP/HFNC without surfactant or intubation are increasingly used. The stress of transfer and the difficulties of close observation during the transport process make non-invasive ventilation more difficult, particularly in the extremely preterm infant. Most infants under 30 weeks should be intubated and given surfactant for transfer. Many teams offer CPAP/HFNC in transport and these may be used if it is appropriate.

Clinical signs of respiratory inadequacy are tachypnea, grunting and recession. Fatigue may be reflected by respiratory pauses or apnoeas. There may be a compensatory tachycardia, with poor perfusion and visible cyanosis.

Monitoring trends in blood gases, oxygen saturations and (where measured) transcutaneous $CO_2$ ($TcCO_2$) and $O_2$ ($TcO_2$) will guide management (Table 14.6).

**Table 14.6** Normal/target values for preterm and term infants

| Parameter | Preterm | Term |
|---|---|---|
| Target temperature | 36–37 °C | 36–37 °C |
| Target $SaO_2$ | 85–93% | >95% (non-cardiac) |
| Target $PaO_2$ | 6–8 kPa (45–60 mmHg) | 8–12 kPa (60–90 mmHg) |
| Target $PaCO_2$ | 4.6–8 kPa (35–60 mmHg) if compensated | 4.6–6.0 kPa (35–45 mmHg) |
| Target blood sugar | >2.6 mmol/l | >2.6 mmol/l |

## Meconium aspiration syndrome

Meconium is typically passed by term babies under stress. If hypoxic and gasping in utero then aspiration may occur. Not all babies who may have aspirated meconium will develop the full blown meconium aspiration syndrome (MAS). MAS causes a pneumonitis; there is a patchy effect with areas of collapse and air trapping. Both pulmonary and cardiac shunting will result in a VQ mismatch. Babies may be affected to a degree that requires ventilatory support. It is likely that the baby will have pulmonary hypertension; if not this may present later and can be very severe. Air trapping can be a problem with risk of air leak (pneumothorax and/or pneumomediastinum). The presence of MAS may indicate fetal distress and there may be a coexisting encephalopathy and other end organ dysfunction (especially myocardial and renal).

If there is respiratory inadequacy then support will be required. The primary problem is usually oxygenation and not $CO_2$ clearance. Air trapping can be very difficult to deal with. Stiff lungs require longer inspiratory times and higher pressure to oxygenate with concomitant risk of air leak. This must be achieved whilst allowing sufficient time for expiration, which may be abnormally long. Surfactant can help, but the effect is sometimes unpredictable and more than two doses may be needed as it is inactivated rapidly by meconium. A high $FiO_2$ can be justified to minimise the risk of persistent pulmonary hypertension of the newborn (PPHN) and encourage pulmonary vasodilatation. This should be titrated to maintain a high normal $PaO_2$. The pH should be maintained at 7.35–7.45 by manipulation of $CO_2$. Sedation with morphine and paralysis with rocuronium or atracurium is vital to minimise pulmonary hypertension.

A significant number of these babies will require high frequency oscillatory ventilation (HFOV) and possibly inhaled nitric oxide to stabilise their condition. Many teams do not offer HFOV en route and the baby will need to be stabilised on a conventional ventilator before transfer. There is strong evidence that babies with severe MAS benefit from management using ECMO and therefore these infants should be discussed with an ECMO centre early on.

Cardiac function may be compromised because of the high ventilatory pressures that are required. The myocardium may also be damaged secondary to hypoxaemia. It is essential to ensure a good cardiac output. Ventilated infants should have arterial access and central venous access secured. Fluid boluses are likely to be required to increase cardiac preload and optimise cardiac output. Inotropic support is usually required in severe cases.

In mature infants it is usual to maintain fluids within the low/restricted range initially (40 ml/kg/day is a typical figure), but hypoglycaemia can be a problem and needs to be managed appropriately.

Systemic blood pressure may need to be maintained at higher than normal levels to overcome high pulmonary pressures in PPHN. A reasonable mean systemic blood pressure in a term infant in these circumstances is 55 mmHg

## Persistent pulmonary hypertension of the newborn

Following birth, all infants have a degree of pulmonary hypertension. In some infants this can cause problems because the pulmonary pressures are so high that they cause a reversal of the normal physiological flow patterns and right–left shunting occurs at intracardiac (foramen ovale) or extracardiac (ductal) levels. Therapeutic strategies are aimed at reversing this. This condition is known variously as PPHN, persistent fetal circulation (PFC) or persistent transitional circulation (PTC). It can occur as an isolated phenomenon following perinatal stress, or can be associated with other problems such as sepsis, MAS or respiratory distress syndrome. Precipitating factors include metabolic acidosis, hypoxia and hypercapnia. Diagnosis should ideally be confirmed by echocardiography. The differential diagnosis of PPHN is that of anomalous pulmonary venous drainage; both result in an enlarged right atrium with reverse shunting but treatment strategies are different.

In general, optimise respiratory and circulatory support and treat any primary conditions if possible.

Ventilatory strategies should aim to maintain oxygenation at high levels to encourage pulmonary vasodilatation. Acidosis will precipitate pulmonary vasoconstriction. Therefore the pH should be maintained 7.35–7.45. This may be achieved through manipulation of $CO_2$. Systemic blood pressure should be maintained with early use of inotropes. The use of selective pulmonary vasodilators may be necessary. If available, nitric oxide should be used. Obviously, if moving a baby who is already on nitric oxide, then the transport system must be capable of maintaining this.

If this is not available, the alternatives that may help include prostacyclin, adenosine or magnesium sulphate. These drugs also have systemic actions and their effect is therefore not predictable. These should only be used by personnel familiar with their actions.

### Circulatory support in the neonatal period

Cardiac function is usually well maintained in preterm infants. Monitoring should be via peripheral arterial line or umbilical artery catheter. If there is evidence of poor perfusion (rising heart rate, increased toe/core temperature gap, skin pallor) then a fluid bolus may be justified to optimise preload and enhance cardiac output. Early consideration should be given to inotropic support.

It is relatively infrequent that the circulation of neonates needs support. They are not usually volume depleted, although in septic conditions, third space losses and reduced vascular tone can manifest as significant intravascular volume depletion. A bolus of 10 ml/kg of fluid may optimise cardiac output.

The ability of the circulation to deliver oxygen is critical. Anaemia reduces the oxygen carrying capacity of the blood. Normal newborn haemoglobins are around 150–160 g/l with haematocrit around 50–60%. A significantly low plasma haemoglobin accompanied by a raised inspired oxygen requirement should prompt consideration of a packed cell transfusion; 15–25 ml/kg of packed cells is likely to increase the haemoglobin by around 40–60 g/l.

Once the circulating volume is optimised then consider inotropic support. The same basic principles apply here as elsewhere. First line drugs used in the neonatal period include dopamine (5–10 micrograms/kg/min) and dobutamine (5–10 micrograms/kg/min). The effects of these drugs are sometimes unpredictable so it is essential to titrate carefully and monitor heart rate, blood pressure, urine output and other signs of perfusion. The aim is to improve cardiac output, not increase blood pressure in isolation. As a rule of thumb the mean blood pressure in mmHg should be greater than or equal to the gestational age in weeks on the first day of life. Low readings without a decrease in urine output and/or metabolic acidosis should probably not be treated.

## 14.8 Surgical problems

### Congenital diaphragmatic hernia

It is increasingly unusual to have to move babies with this condition long distances after birth. The majority are diagnosed antenatally and electively delivered in or very close to a specialist surgical centre. However, even within a surgical centre these infants will need moving between intensive care and theatre.

Problems arise due to pulmonary hypoplasia (especially on the side of the hernia), the presence of abdominal contents in the thoracic cavity and associated pulmonary hypertension. Intubation should be performed as soon as possible to permit lung inflation without gastric distension, which may occur with bag–valve–mask support. This is especially true as the lungs may have poor compliance and be quite stiff to bag. Such distension may further compromise breathing because of the effect of the distended gut compressing the lung tissue.

High ventilation pressures with long inspiratory times may be required. There is a significant risk of air leak in this situation. Pneumothoraces will require prompt drainage. Surfactant may be helpful in optimising alveolar recruitment. HFOV is a very effective mode of ventilation in these infants and should be used if it is available. When this is not possible, infants already on HFOV must be converted from this mode prior to any move. This transition should occur long enough before the move to confirm stability. A nasogastric (NG) tube should be passed early to minimise gastric distension. It should be aspirated regularly and left on free drainage between times. Target values for gas exchange are to keep the $PaO_2$ in the high normal range, pH around 7.35–7.45 and $PaCO_2$ in the low normal range to maintain the pH. This will maximise pulmonary vasodilatation and minimise any tendency to PPHN. Sedation and paralysis will usually be required in ventilated babies.

Full monitoring with arterial access is essential. Maintenance fluids should be provided with 10% dextrose. If there is evidence of pulmonary hypertension appropriate strategies should be employed. Additional boluses of fluid, early inotropic support and nitric oxide may be required.

Babies with a congenital diaphragmatic hernia may have associated cardiac defects. Ideally an echocardiogram should be performed to assess the presence or absence of these prior to transfer.

## Oesophageal atresia/tracheo-oesophageal fistula

These are often identified antenatally (during investigation of polyhydramnios), but may also be diagnosed postnatally following cyanotic or aspiration episodes. With oesophageal atresia problems arise because the infant cannot swallow their own saliva. It then pools and may be aspirated. Where there is a coexisting fistula, respiratory difficulties may be compounded by gaseous distension of the stomach. This may cause vagal overactivity and splinting of the diaphragm that can even precipitate a cardiac arrest. It is anatomically impossible to aspirate the stomach and therefore this tendency must be minimised. Decompression and aspiration of any proximal pouch should be undertaken.

A replogle tube under continuous suction should be used to remove accumulating secretions (Figure 14.1). Where possible, these infants should be allowed to breathe spontaneously. Positive pressure ventilation should be avoided wherever possible, when there is a tracheo-oesophageal fistula (TOF), as the stomach is more distensible than the lungs (particularly in the preterm infant) and gastric distension causes splinting of the chest. Gastric rupture can also occur.

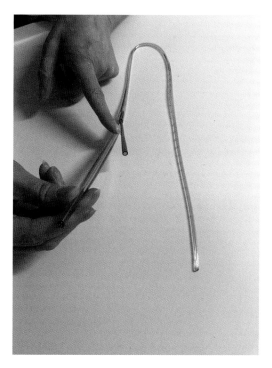

**Figure 14.1  Replogle tube.** Courtesy of Cassie Lawn

The cardiovascular system and circulation do not usually present a problem. There may be associated cardiac defects, which should ideally be identified/excluded prior to any move. Maintenance fluids should be administered intravenously at normal rates.

It is important to note that the common abbreviation TOF may also be used for the cardiac abnormality tetralogy of Fallot. It is therefore recommended that both of these conditions are always given their unabbreviated names.

## Exomphalos/gastroschisis

Exomphalos (herniation of the abdominal contents into the umbilical cord) and gastroschisis (herniation of the abdominal contents through an abdominal wall defect beside the umbilical cord) require similar approaches. Gastroschisis requires a more urgent transfer to a surgical unit. However, it is important to note that exomphalos is much more frequently associated with other congenital abnormalities. Both of these lesions are usually diagnosed on antenatal ultrasound examinations.

Airway and breathing are not usually a problem. Most infants do not require support unless there are other coexisting problems.

The circulation may require support. Fluid losses from the exposed abdominal contents may be significant (especially with a gastroschisis, where the intestines are exposed). It is important to ensure that there is adequate venous access (preferably one central and one peripheral line). Maintenance fluids of 60–90 ml/kg/day should be given to maintain blood glucose. Boluses of fluid are almost always required in gastroschisis to replace high insensible losses. It is good practice to review this requirement and increase maintenance fluid to cover these losses. An increasing metabolic acidosis or rising lactate must be investigated with diligence as it may indicate bowel ischaemia.

Treatment priorities are to protect the bowel from damage and minimise heat and fluid loss. The bowel may be wrapped in cling film to reduce evaporative and convective heat loss. The bowel should be positioned and covered to prevent it twisting on its pedicle, which could compromise the vascular supply. In a transport incubator, the infant may typically be nursed on their side. The clear material also allows a regular visual inspection of the bowel.

An NG tube should be inserted and aspirated regularly as distension of the bowel could cause mechanical effects and tension on the vascular pedicle. Compromised bowel may appear dusky or even black and should prompt urgent action. It is wise to discuss the care of these babies with a paediatric surgeon, especially if bowel viability is in question.

Exomphalos may be associated with other conditions such as Beckwith–Weiderman syndrome. These hyperinsulinaemic infants are at high risk of hypoglycaemia, which must be identified and treated aggressively. Increased fluid volumes, higher concentrations of dextrose and occasionally glucagon may be required.

## Gastrointestinal obstruction

Gastrointestinal obstruction may occur as part of a number of congenital conditions or as a consequence of other problems. Small and large bowel atresias, malrotation or meconium ileus may all present with a distended abdomen, failure to tolerate feeds, vomiting, discomfort or more significant problems arising as a result of secondary compromise to the gut, or of electrolyte disturbance.

A suspected malrotation and volvulus should be considered a time critical transfer. In some cases bowel distension may splint the diaphragm and cause respiratory embarrassment. There are also risks of vomiting and aspiration. Stopping enteral intake is mandatory. Decompression via an NG tube may reduce distension and will reduce the chance of aspiration.

If there has been significant vomiting or other fluid loss then the circulation may be compromised and resuscitation fluids may be required. Intravenous access is essential with adequate fluid to replace any deficit and to keep up with maintenance requirements and any continuing losses. If there have been significant NG losses, then there may be electrolyte disturbance as a result. Sodium and potassium losses can be significant. NG aspirates should be replaced with normal saline with added potassium.

## Necrotising enterocolitis

Necrotising enterocolitis (NEC) is a condition which is most common in preterm babies. The abdomen distends, the baby stops tolerating enteral feeds and may have bilious vomiting or aspirates. If an X-ray is taken it may show pathognomonic features such as intramural gas or gas in the biliary tree. The bowel inflammation is associated with marked changes in bowel wall permeability and there may be marked fluid loss into the bowel. All infants should be nil by mouth with a wide bore NG tube in situ on free drainage and receive broad-spectrum antibiotics.

Where the abdomen is significantly distended, ventilation may be required due to respiratory compromise. Relatively high pressures may be needed in response to the diaphragmatic splinting. An NG tube should be passed and maintained on continuous drainage to minimise the intraluminal volume.

Fluid resuscitation may be required if fluid loss into the bowel has been significant. There may be thrombocytopenia and even disseminated intravascular coagulation in severe cases.

Many babies who are initially treated as possibly having NEC resolve rapidly with medical intervention. The presence of NEC may be uncertain in these cases. However, some babies do have definite disease and it is routine to keep these babies nil by mouth (and hence needing total parental nutrition) for 7–14 days. Such babies may need transfer to a surgical centre for insertion of a central line (usually semi-electively). In more serious cases, a surgical referral is made for bowel perforation with or without evidence of peritonitis. Such babies may appear relatively well, or may be in extremis and can present significant challenges to the transfer team.

## 14.9 Summary

This chapter summarises the important physiological differences between infants and small children and adults. A structured ABCDEF approach to the primary survey during the transfer process has been outlined. This initial assessment must be followed by a secondary survey including consideration of the most appropriate destination for ongoing care according to likely diagnosis. Some key considerations when managing some specific conditions have also been outlined.

# CHAPTER 15
# Clinical considerations for adults

---

### Learning outcomes

After reading this chapter, you will be able to:
- Describe how the systematic ACCEPT approach enables movements of ill and injured patients between or within hospitals

---

## 15.1 Introduction

Each day in the UK, a variety of seriously ill and injured patients are transported within or between hospitals. The systematic ACCEPT approach enables these movements to be carried out safely and effectively. In previous chapters the components of ACCEPT have been described followed by an overview of the clinical aspects of the ABCDEF approach to medicine.

In the past, many transfers of critically ill patients were dictated by the lack of critical care facilities at the transferring centre. The expansion of level 2 and level 3 facilities and the development of local resource escalation policies have resulted in a reduction in the number of these non-clinical transfers.

Specialist services are being centralised and regionalised so that now patients are transferred to address very specific clinical needs. In this chapter some of these broad categories of patients will be considered, based on the types of specialist centres, and their specific transfer challenges.

- Neurosurgery
  - Traumatic brain injury
  - Cerebral bleeds
- Trauma
- Burns
- Vascular surgery
  - Abdominal aortic aneurysm (AAA)
  - Thoracic aortic dissection
  - Acute limb ischaemia
- Interventional radiology
- Cardiology
  - Primary coronary intervention
- Nephrology
  - Acute renal failure
- Obstetric
- Level 3 transfers

---

*Neonatal, Adult and Paediatric Safe Transfer and Retrieval: A Practical Approach to Transfers*, First Edition.
Edited by Bernard Foëx, Peter-Marc Fortune and Cassie Lawn.
© 2019 John Wiley & Sons Ltd. Published 2019 by John Wiley & Sons Ltd.

## 15.2 Transfer of the neurosurgical patient

Inter-hospital transfer of the patient with traumatic and non-traumatic brain injury to a tertiary centre is both common and challenging. These transfers are often relatively time critical, involve patients with significant morbidity and require careful management of raised intracranial pressure (ICP).

Examples of neurosurgical problems requiring patient transfer include:

- Traumatic brain injury
- Subarachnoid haemorrhage
- Intracranial haemorrhage
- Brain abscess

---

**General principles**

- Seek early advice from a tertiary referral centre
- Position the patient at approximately 30° head-up (unless a coexisting cervical spine injury precludes this) and ensure the endotracheal tube ties are not too tight. These measures help with the prevention of venous congestion and may contribute to the management of raised ICP
- Maintain close scrutiny of the Glasgow Coma Scale (GCS) and pupillary response to light by regular systematic examination

---

### Airway

The airway should be secured with a cuffed oral endotracheal tube in the following situations:

- GCS score <9
- Labile or deteriorating GCS score, even when greater than 9
- Severe agitation, making the transfer unsafe for the patient and/or crew
- When the injury is significant and the transfer time prolonged
- When the accepting team advise intubation

Given the complexity of these patients and the potential need for the management of raised ICP, a low threshold for intubation and ventilation should be maintained.

### Breathing

Avoid hypoxia in brain-injured patients.

Aim for a $PaO_2 > 10$ kPa.

In the ventilated patient ensure normocarbia ($PaCO_2$ 4.5–5 kPa) and consider hyperventilation ($PaCO_2$ 4–4.5 kPa) if raised ICP is suspected.

### Circulation

Avoid hypotension. Aim for a mean arterial pressure of at least 90 mmHg with the aim of preserving cerebral perfusion.

An arterial line should be placed to allow accurate beat-to-beat monitoring of blood pressure. Consider central venous access, if time allows.

Vasopressors may be required to achieve mean arterial pressure goals.

Correct any coagulopathy.

Careful use of intravenous fluid may be needed to achieve euvolaemia and normal plasma sodium and lactate levels.

## Disability

Maintain normothermia and blood glucose levels below 10 mmol/l.

Avoid pyrexia and start warming measures if shivering occurs to avoid increasing oxygen demand.

## Specific conditions

### *Traumatic brain injury*

Management focuses on the avoidance of secondary brain injury by controlling the ICP and maintaining cerebral perfusion pressure.

Initial measures include:

- Secure the airway if indicated (see earlier in this chapter)
- Position to 30° head-up and avoid tight endotracheal tube ties
- Avoid hypotension and hypoxaemia
- Maintain blood sugar <10 mmol/l

> **If raised or rising ICP is suspected then consider the following interventions. These are best carried out in a tertiary neurosurgical centre and advice should be sought before commencing these prior to transfer.**

- Ventilate to normocarbia ($pCO_2$ 4.5–5 kPa)
- Deepen sedation and consider neuromuscular blockade early
- Maintain mean arterial pressure >90 mmHg; use vasopressors if necessary, metaraminol may be used in time critical situations where central venous catheter placement and commencement of noradrenaline may be too time consuming
- Treat seizures with anticonvulsant therapy
- Osmotherapy may be considered, for example:
  - Mannitol 10% (about 200 ml bolus for 70 kg adult)
  - Mannitol 20% (about 100 ml bolus for 70 kg adult)
  - Hypertonic saline (15 ml 30% NaCl over 10 minutes via a central line)
- If there is a suspicion that these measures are failing (e.g. blown pupil, non-reassuring computed tomography scan) consider boluses and/or infusion of barbiturates and therapeutic hypothermia

### *Subarachnoid haemorrhage*

This is a relatively common and often devastating condition. Patients with aneurysmal subarachnoid haemorrhage (SAH) should be considered as emergency cases; the risk of rebleeding within the first 24 hours is high. Aneurysms are treated radiologically or surgically by coiling or clipping at a tertiary centre. Evacuation of haematoma, insertion of an extraventricular drain or craniectomy may also be needed.

A sudden increase in ICP is often seen in SAH and treatment should follow the general principles outlined earlier. Cardiorespiratory complications, such as myocardial dysfunction and pulmonary oedema, may follow, provoked by a catecholamine surge as a result of the injury. These should be treated if they arise. Definitive treatment will not be possible prior to transfer but haemodynamic stability should be sought after definitive airway protection and treatment of raised ICP. Aim for a systolic blood pressure <180 mmHg in patients with an unprotected (untreated) aneurysm.

### *Intracranial haemorrhage*

Recent trial evidence has recommended that blood pressure management with intravenous agents, such as an infusion of labetalol, should be considered when:

- Presentation is within 6 hours of onset and systolic blood pressure is >150 mmHg. Aim for a systolic blood pressure <140 mmHg in these patients
- Presentation is after 6 hours from symptom onset and systolic blood pressure is >200 mmHg. Aim for a systolic blood pressure <180 mmHg in these patients

Note: the above guidelines do not apply to known or suspected aneurysmal SAH. Seek advice from the tertiary centre in these patients

## 15.3 Transfer of the trauma patient

The advent of major trauma centres (MTCs) has greatly changed trauma care. Most major trauma patients are now taken directly to MTCs rather than the nearest hospital. However, there is still scope for major trauma patients being taken to a trauma unit for stabilisation of an impending airway problem or because they did not appear critically injured at first. These patients will be transferred on to the MTC for definitive treatment.

---

**General principles**

A   Airway (burns: stabilise early – uncut tube)
B   Ventilation (chest drains, escharotomy, positive end expiratory pressure (PEEP) for flail segments)
C   Circulation (fluid resuscitation/transfusion/blood products, burns fluids, tranexamic acid, urinary catheter)
D   Sedation/analgesia
E   Temperature – avoid hypothermia because of coagulopathy
F   Family

---

## 15.4 Transfer of the burns patient

Transfer criteria to specialist centres may include:

- >20% body surface area (BSA)
- >10% BSA in the elderly
- >5% BSA full thickness
- Chemical burns
- Inhalation injury
- Burns to special areas (face, eyes, ears, perineum, genitalia, flexures over joints)
- Significant electrical burns

### Airway

An inhalational injury, which may result in airway compromise, should be suspected when you find:

- Peri-oral burns
- Singed eyebrows/nasal hair
- Soot in mouth
- Soot in sputum
- Pharyngeal erythema/blistering
- Hoarse voice or stridor
- High oxygen requirement
- High carboxyhaemoglobin

Intubation should be considered early as airway oedema may develop quickly. If there is already upper airway oedema plan for a possible surgical airway, in case oral intubation is impossible.

Always use an uncut endotracheal tube to accommodate facial swelling.

### Breathing

Consider escharotomy in a circumferential chest burn to prevent ventilatory compromise en route.

### Circulation

Secure intravenous access is needed (ideally not through burned tissue).

Fluid management should be agreed with the burns unit, usually based on the patient's weight and BSA burned.

Monitor urine output (aim for 1 ml/kg/h).

## Disability

Sedation and analgesia, if the patient is ventilated. If not intubated and ventilated, adequate analgesia will be needed.

Large BSA burns may be associated with nausea, vomiting and gastric distension. Consider antiemetics and passing a nasogastric tube before transfer.

## Exposure

Check for other injuries, for example 'escape' injuries or injuries caused by falling masonry.

Circumferential burns – discuss possible need for escharotomy with the burns unit before transfer (not usually needed in the first few hours).

## 15.5 Transfer of the vascular surgery patient

### Abdominal aortic aneurysm

Bleeding from a ruptured AAA, or other aneurysmal rupture, carries a very high risk of death. The life-saving intervention is specialist surgery or an endovascular aneurysm repair (EVAR). This will require transfer to a specialist vascular surgery centre.

---

**General principles**
- These are generally time critical transfers
- Once the diagnosis is made, keep stabilisation to a minimum
- Do not wait for blood products
- As the definitive treatment is surgery a medical escort is unlikely to add value to the transfer team

---

### Thoracic aortic dissection

This is a rare condition. Management should be discussed with the specialist centre before transfer. This may include management of blood pressure.

### Acute limb ischaemia

In the case of a traumatic ischaemic limb it will be necessary to stabilise life-threatening injuries before transfer.

Peripheral vascular disease patients will usually not need ABC stabilisation but may need stabilisation of other complications of their underlying problem, for example, diabetes.

## 15.6 Transfer of the patient for interventional radiology

Interventional radiology is increasingly being used as an alternative to emergency surgery in a number of surgical and medical causes of haemorrhage. However, this is only available in specialist centres. Patients being transferred to these centres may be time critical, for example bleeding from a ruptured AAA, or may be intensive, for example an intubated patient being transferred from an intensive care unit (ICU) for a transjugular intrahepatic portosystemic shunt (TIPS) after immediate management of bleeding oesophageal varices.

The following are patients who may need transfer for interventional radiology.

### Trauma

- Liver lacerations
- Pelvic injuries

## Surgical

- Aneurysm ruptures
- Ischaemic limbs
- Lower gastrointestinal haemorrhage

## Medical

- Upper gastrointestinal haemorrhage
- Oesophageal/gastric varices
- TIPS

## 15.7 Transfer of the cardiology patient

Now that paramedic ambulances carry electrocardiogram (ECG) machines most out-of-hospital ST elevation myocardial infarctions (STEMIs) are diagnosed on scene and patients are transferred directly to cardiology centres for immediate assessment, usually involving angiography and primary coronary intervention (PCI) to reperfuse ischaemic myocardium.

Patients who self-present with a STEMI and those who suffer a STEMI as in-patients in hospitals without interventional facilities will need to be transferred to their local centre.

---

**General principles**

- These are time critical transfers

---

Most patients will not need any form of stabilisation, in which case a paramedic crew can transfer them. Their principal risk is a cardiac arrest en route. Paramedics have the skills and generally have much more experience at managing out-of-hospital cardiac arrests than hospital staff, so there may be little 'added value' in having a medical escort for the transfer.

Most patients will not need any airway protection or ventilatory or cardiac support. In rare instances (for example in cardiogenic shock) patients may need stabilisation with vasopressors, in which case a medical escort will be needed.

Hospitals without interventional cardiology services will be paired with their local centre. There should be agreed transfer criteria and guidance on any pre-transfer stabilisation or drug treatments. This is likely to include the use of aspirin and other specific antiplatelet treatments.

## 15.8 Transfer of the patient with acute renal failure

Patients in acute renal failure may need urgent renal replacement treatment because of fluid overload, hyperkalaemia, uraemic encephalopathy or a combination of these complications. Most ICUs will be able to provide some sort of renal replacement, even if there are no haemodialysis facilities, to allow immediate stabilisation of the patient before transfer to a dialysis centre for ongoing management.

In those cases when this is not possible, the patient will need to be transferred.

### Fluid overload

If the patient is in respiratory failure as a consequence of fluid overload non-invasive ventilation may be used to stabilise the patient before transfer. If this fails invasive ventilation and an intensive level transfer may be needed.

### Hyperkalaemia

This must be managed before transfer. Intravenous calcium is used for cardiac stabilisation. This can be followed by an infusion of insulin and dextrose to promote intracellular movement of potassium and salbutamol nebulisers.

## Uraemia

If the patient is encephalopathic, then the airway must be protected. Intubation and ventilation and an intensive level transfer will be necessary. Patients with uraemia severe enough to cause encephalopathy may also have a pericardial effusion and may show signs of cardiac compromise. Echocardiography should be performed before transfer to establish whether this is the case. Drainage of the effusion and/or inotropic/vasopressor support can then be considered as part of the stabilisation process before transfer.

## 15.9 Transfer of the obstetric patient

For the purposes of this section, obstetric patient means a patient who is pregnant. An obstetric patient is usually transferred for expert management of the sick *mother* or for the in utero transfer of the sick or premature *fetus* to a unit with neonatal intensive care facilities. It may be safer to deliver the baby before transfer in this situation.

---

**General principles**

- The decision to transfer an obstetric patient should be made at consultant level
- Ensure that in addition to obstetric and midwifery staff, paediatricians, obstetric anaesthetists and intensivists (if necessary) have all been informed of and agree to the transfer, both in the referring and receiving hospitals
- It is important to know exactly where the patient is to be transferred to in the receiving hospital. Some hospitals have a high dependency unit within the delivery suite – double check the exact location of the receiving area

---

### Airway

Securing the airway of the pregnant patient in later pregnancy can be difficult because of the anatomical changes that occur.

### Breathing

Breathing may be embarrassed by similar changes in anatomy; there is an increased risk of aspiration pneumonitis due to poor gastric emptying, and a tendency for gastric reflux to occur.

### Circulation

Pregnant women after 25–30 weeks' gestation should not be nursed supine because aorto-caval compression can compromise both the mother's and baby's circulation. The use of a wedge under the right hip will help to reduce this problem; however, the tilting of the patient may reduce accessibility to the patient in an ambulance (Figure 15.1).

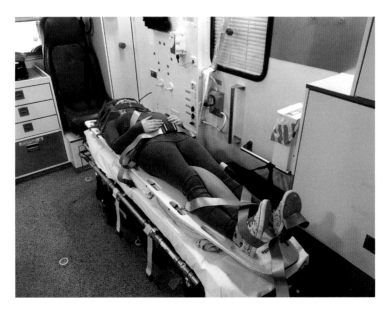

**Figure 15.1 Tilting an obstetric patient.** Courtesy of Matthew Davis

## Specific conditions

### Pre-eclampsia and eclampsia

This tends to occur in the third trimester of pregnancy. It is characterised by hypertension and proteinuria. Left untreated it may progress to seizures, when it is defined as eclampsia. Definitive treatment is delivery of the fetus and placenta. Timing of the delivery is a balance between minimising the risk of complications for the mother and the risks associated with premature delivery for the baby.

Management of blood pressure may be necessary using drugs such as labetalol, hydralazine or nifedipine. Magnesium sulphate may be needed to reduce the risk of seizures. These management decisions should be made in consultation with the specialist obstetric unit before transfer. Patients managed with an intravenous infusion of an antihypertensive should be monitored with an arterial line and should have central venous access before transfer.

### Eclampsia

This condition occurs when a pre-eclamptic patient develops new seizures with no alternative aetiology. It carries a high risk of perinatal and maternal mortality and morbidity. Intravenous magnesium sulphate should be used to prevent and treat seizures. Intravenous anticonvulsants should be used if magnesium sulphate is ineffective.

Airway management and invasive ventilation may be needed as part of seizure management.

Blood pressure management will be needed as for pre-eclampsia.

## 15.10 Level 3 transfers: the complex ICU patient

These are critically ill patients, often needing multi-organ support, who need to be transferred from one ICU to another for specialist management of one of their organ failures. Examples of conditions in such patients would be severe respiratory failure/acute respiratory distress syndrome (ARDS) needing specific treatments such as extracorporeal membrane oxygenation, severe pancreatitis and acute liver failure.

### Airway

The airway should be secured.

### Breathing

The transport ventilator can replicate pre-transfer settings, especially a high PEEP and 1:1 or inverse ratio ventilation, which may be needed in severe ARDS.

Ensure the patient is settled on the transport ventilator well before transfer to allow time to check blood gases and ensure adequate oxygenation and ventilation. Monitor the end-tidal $CO_2$. Calculate the oxygen requirements for the transfer.

### Circulation

Piggyback vasopressor infusions, including a contingency plan with a vasopressor that can be delivered peripherally, such as metaraminol.

Monitor the urine output.

If dialysis or renal replacement therapy (RRT) dependent, provide a clear handover of the last dialysis session or when RRT was discontinued prior to transfer and plan likely dialysis/RRT needs on arrival.

### Disability/Dextrose

Ensure there is adequate sedation and paralysis, including a contingency plan to use bolus doses in case of infusion pump failure.

**Environment**

Avoid hypothermia – pre-warm the ambulance, mummy-wrap the patient and use a hat to reduce heat loss.

**Family**

Ensure appropriate communications are maintained with the family at all times.

## 15.11  Summary

Centralisation of specialist services means more transfers for clinical reasons.

Many of these transfers will be time critical, some will be intensive, and some will be both. This chapter has provided an overview of the patient groups that typically will need to be transferred to specialist centres, some of their characteristics and associated specific clinical management.

However, early and effective communication between centres is essential to ensure that any specific treatments are administered before or during the transfer to optimise patient care.

# PART 5
# Special considerations

# CHAPTER 16
# Support for the family

---

## Learning outcomes

After reading this chapter, you will be able to:
- Discuss the importance of regular, clear communication with family members, throughout the transfer process

---

## 16.1 Introduction

The transfer of a critically ill patient can be a very difficult time for families. It is not uncommon that the situation has progressed from that of having a normal, healthy mother, father, brother, sister, child, etc. or expecting a healthy baby, to one of having a critically ill family member receiving intensive care. Even if the condition is not life threatening it may often appear so to the family. They will be stressed and frightened. They may also be very tired. On occasions these factors may manifest as anger. It is vital that the clinical team recognise this and do not react and reflect anger back.

## 16.2 Communications by the transfer team

Communication should be clear, honest, open and concise. Speculation and unrealistic assurances must be avoided. The need to transfer a critically ill patient may not have been anticipated by the family. With regards to children and neonates, this transfer may be to a hospital far from their home. The reasons for the transfer should be explained with great care to avoid undermining parental confidence in their local centre. This is key as the patient, and especially so if a child, may return to their local care in the future. Wherever possible, informed consent for the transfer should be sought. This can be verbal but it is important to follow your own trust/services guidelines.

Communications with families should be undertaken by the most appropriate member of the attending team wherever possible. Honesty is vital throughout the process, with the risks and benefits of transfer being openly discussed. Family members should be offered the opportunity to travel with the patient, space permitting, and should be actively encouraged especially when the child is conscious.

This chapter will focus on family support (Figure 16.1) in terms of:

- Before the transfer
- During the transfer
- After the transfer
- Respecting family wishes
- Consent for transfer

## 16.3 Before the transfer

On arrival the transfer team should introduce themselves to the patient's family. Detailed discussions are usually better deferred until after the team has had a clinical handover and an opportunity to clinically assess the patient. Giving the family some indication of the timing of such discussions can be helpful.

---

*Neonatal, Adult and Paediatric Safe Transfer and Retrieval: A Practical Approach to Transfers*, First Edition.
Edited by Bernard Foëx, Peter-Marc Fortune and Cassie Lawn.
© 2019 John Wiley & Sons Ltd. Published 2019 by John Wiley & Sons Ltd.

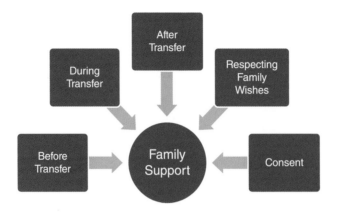

**Figure 16.1 Family support**

> **Do not underestimate the work you have to do in this regard.**

Once you are fully appraised of the clinical situation, a more detailed discussion may be undertaken with the family. It is vital that before this discussion you are aware of previous conversations that the family have had with the local team and what they have understood. This might be best facilitated by asking them what they have already been told. Even the most informed of relatives may erroneously process information at times of stress and anxiety. Therefore, their understanding may be at considerable variance to the content of the conversation as described by the local team. In very complex situations, just the sheer volume of information can be bewildering. Expectations from previous conversations may need to be carefully managed especially in an evolving clinical setting. Furthermore, it is not uncommon for relatives to feel that once a transfer team arrives 'everything is going to be fine'. Once again, any need to revise a prognosis downward should be handled without inadvertent criticism of local care.

It is quite natural to want to reassure family members but honesty is vital. Any reassurance must be done within the limits of the patient's likely outcome. In grave situations inappropriate optimism may give false hope which will make later management very difficult. This is especially true where a withdrawal of advanced support becomes appropriate.

In paediatric cases, most families will wish to accompany their children on a transfer. There is no standard guidance as to whether they should or not, but they should be actively encouraged to do so. Whether it is possible depends on many factors. Local team policy will influence this, as will practical issues around space, the child's clinical status and mode of transfer. Wherever possible, a member of the family should accompany a conscious child so as to minimise the child's distress. The fact that a child has a significant risk of dying during the transfer should not prevent their relative accompanying them. In fact it might be that on these occasions there are very powerful arguments to support their presence. The time taken to transfer the child may be a significant part of a child's remaining life and family should never be excluded. Furthermore, should the child die en route, the presence of the family member may make their acceptance and understanding of the situation easier.

Mothers of newborn infants should not accompany them on transfer unless the mother is medically fit to do so, i.e. has been discharged from hospital care, or there is a midwife to care for the mother during transfer. This is rarely possible as there is insufficient space in the back of an ambulance for a mother, a midwife and adult resuscitation equipment as well as a neonatal transport incubator, equipment and team. Many teams have developed local guidelines to support this and these should be referred to.

When relatives travel with the transport team it is vital to discuss 'ground rules' before setting off. It must be made clear that should a significant deterioration take place the family member must allow the team unhindered access to the patient and their equipment. In an aircraft they will usually be in a seat somewhat separated from their relative which they must stay in. On road ambulance transfers they should be advised that they will be required to remain seated, or to vacate the back of the ambulance to allow the team to work. Very careful consideration should be given to allowing agitated or aggressive relatives to travel with the team.

Many transfer teams carry hospital information packs for their regional units, with contact numbers, maps and travel information. It is helpful if these can be given to family members prior to their relative's departure to enable them to plan their journey if they are not going to travel with the transfer team, or to pass the information on to other family members if they are. Clear information regarding how and when to reach their relative at the receiving centre is helpful. If at all possible, transport should be arranged for the family that does not involve them driving. If they do drive, gentle, non-patronising advice should be given regarding their driving style – they should be advised not to try to 'chase the ambulance' as this is both dangerous and illegal.

It is good practice to ensure that family members do not leave the referring hospital before the transport team. There have been a number of incidents where the patient has deteriorated or even died prior to departure of the retrieval team, but after the family had left. The family then arrives at the receiving centre to be given the terrible information by an unfamiliar team, only to have to return to the referring hospital to be with their relative.

## 16.4 During the transfer

It is not always possible or appropriate to contact family members during a transfer, however a brief update, even if only via a text, is greatly appreciated by families, especially if it is a long transfer. This is usually non-clinical information – e.g. safe arrival. Detailed clinical information is best reserved for face-to-face communications.

If family members travel with the team caring for them is also important. They are most likely very tired and stressed. Offering to charge their mobile phone if the ambulance has 240V power sockets, allowing them to stay in touch with other family members, will be gratefully received. They may also not have eaten or had a drink for some time and having snack packs on board for them can be most comforting.

## 16.5 After the transfer

Most teams will communicate with family members at the completion of a transfer, not only to say how the transfer went but also to give specific information regarding their relative's exact location in the new facility, as well as contact names and numbers of the new medical/nursing team.

If there has been open and honest discussion before and during the transfer a poor outcome should not come as a bolt from the blue. This will not reduce the impact of bad news but being poorly prepared may worsen distress. In the event of an unexpected adverse incident the same principles of clear, open and honest communication that should underpin the whole transfer process still apply. If the patient dies before the family arrives it will usually be better to wait for face-to-face contact rather than contacting them en route.

## 16.6 Respecting family wishes

Family wishes and expectations should always be treated with the utmost respect. If there appears to be a disparity between the clinical needs of the patient, as perceived by the transfer team, and family wishes this must be promptly referred to the consultant in charge for urgent consideration and direction.

Cultural and religious views should also be considered when talking to family. Where possible a qualified interpreter should be sought if English is not the family's first language.

## 16.7 Consent for transfer

Most transfers of critically ill patients take place with no more than verbal consent from the family. On rare occasions family members may raise an objection to transfer. This will usually be because they do not believe it is in their relative's best interests. This is most likely to arise because of a lack of understanding of the need for transfer. It will usually be resolved by further discussion and explanation of key issues.

It is possible that a family member may refuse to agree to their relative being transferred even after lengthy discussions. In these circumstances, if the patient is at risk of significant harm from not being transferred, it may be acceptable to do so against the relative's wishes. The most senior member of the transfer team must be involved in the decision-making process and a clear written record must be kept of all discussions and reasons for decisions that are made. Relatives must be kept informed of any decision taken against their wishes and the reasons for those decisions. It is sometimes helpful in these circumstances to involve other family members or religious/pastoral leaders in these discussions.

In the case of a paediatric patient any safeguarding concerns will need to be documented and handed over to the referring team accepting the care of the child.

Specific consent may be needed from parents for procedures that are planned at the receiving centre, e.g. extracorporeal membrane oxygenation or surgery. If a parent is not accompanying a child on a transfer this can be a problem. If the procedure cannot wait for a face-to-face meeting then usual practice would be for the clinician carrying out the procedure to obtain verbal consent over the telephone. It is helpful to warn parents this may happen and to ensure that the transfer team has the relevant contact information.

Children over 16, or those less than 16 years of age who are deemed competent to understand the risks and benefits of a procedure, may give consent to their own treatment. However, children in acute transfer situations are usually too unwell to do so. Children without parents or those in state care can have consent given by a legal guardian or parent who holds parental responsibility. Both parents can give consent to treatment of their child if they are married. Unmarried fathers can only give consent if they are named on the child's birth certificate, have formally adopted the child or have been given parental responsibility by the courts. This can be an issue in newborn infants before registration of the birth. If the mother has just given birth and remains an in-patient it is important to obtain the mother's contact number if the child is not registered to allow verbal consent to be taken for any procedure over the phone. Further information regarding consent issues can be found on the General Medical Council website at www.gmc-uk.org.

## 16.8 Summary

In this chapter we have highlighted the importance of clear, open, honest and concise communication with family members throughout the transfer process. This underpins the establishment of a trusting relationship with them, which may help to minimise distress at an extremely difficult time. Preparing critically ill patients and their families with honest clinical information as well as practical information will help them to regain some control in what can be an extremely frightening situation.

# CHAPTER 17
# Air transfers – an introduction

---

### Learning outcomes

After reading this chapter, you will be able to:
- Explain the benefits and disadvantages of aeromedical transfer
- Recognise the importance of the structured approach to aviation transfer medicine
- Appreciate the unique safety issues encountered in aeromedical transfers

---

## 17.1 Introduction

Aeromedical transportation may be undertaken by aeroplane (fixed wing) or helicopter (rotary wing) aircraft. This distinction is useful, as each broad type of aircraft has its own set of advantages and challenges in terms of the aeromedical working environment.

Generally, air transport should be reserved for longer journeys or for journeys over water. Fixed-wing aircraft, preferably pressurised, should be considered for transfer distances of more than 150 miles (240 km). It is important to remember that the perceived speed of air transfer must be balanced against organisational delays, inter-vehicle transfers and loading/unloading at either end of the journey.

Air transfers are usually undertaken for one of the following reasons: to shorten the time taken to access an expert team or to access definitive care, to minimise the duration of time that an unstable patient is outside a hospital environment, or when consumables (e.g. oxygen) make road transport inappropriate.

Most aeromedical activity is delivered by private companies providing repatriation services, helicopter emergency medical services (HEMS) providing 'scene' response (pre-hospital care), or dedicated critical care retrieval teams.

## 17.2 Helicopter transfers

The use of helicopters for the transfer of patients has been the subject of some debate. The transfer of patients by helicopter has advantages in sparsely populated areas or in a maritime environment. In this kind of environment, a helicopter can deliver medical, nursing or paramedical teams enabling on scene resuscitation to proceed. However, in an urban environment, helicopters may have no advantage over a well equipped road-based service (see References and further reading).

Most helicopters used for medical transfers in the UK have the following limitations:

- Limited range without refuelling
- Limited cargo weight
- Flying frequently restricted because of weather conditions
- Lack of availability of landing places
- Often require road transfers at the beginning and end of each fight
- En route therapeutic interventions are limited by space.
- Cabin environment is noisy making monitoring and communication difficult
- High running costs

---

Road transportation has the following advantages:

- Healthcare staff are more familiar with this environment
- Rapid mobilisation time
- Transfer is usually door to door
- Patient monitoring and observation are easier
- Vehicle can be halted to undertake therapeutic interventions
- Vehicle can be easily diverted
- Minimal disruption from adverse weather conditions
- Lower overall cost

### Civil air ambulances

In the UK, there are currently 18 civil air ambulance services, undertaking approximately 125 000 'scene calls' per year. Heart attack victims and 'collapsed' patients in remote areas also make up a significant proportion of the workload. Air ambulance helicopter services are classed as civil operations; they are usually charitably funded and are organised by private organisations. These are in turn contracted by an NHS ambulance trust. The scope of work undertaken by air ambulances is limited by the following:

- Funding
- Availability of aircraft or pilots
- Range
- Weather

In general, in England and Wales, civil charitable air ambulance operations are restricted to daylight hours because the aircraft have to find a landing site visually when they arrive at the scene. It is possible to operate from designated helipads after dark provided that these are suitably lit either from the ground or from the helicopter. There is known to be a significant increase in helicopter accidents during night-time missions and in poor weather conditions.

### Search and rescue medtransfer assistance

The Maritime and Coastguard Agency maintains a year-round, 24-hour search and rescue service covering the whole of the UK and a large part of the surrounding sea. The service has been tendered and will be delivered by Bristow helicopters. The service will consider assisting with rotary wing aeromedical transfers in an emergency and should be contacted via the local statutory ambulance provider.

### Arranging a helicopter transfer

Air ambulance and HEMS may be available free to the NHS, through funding supported by charitable donations. However, any cost should be identified as early as possible along with an agreement to pay from the appropriate budget holder. Search and rescue assistance is expensive. The requesting hospital NHS trust will be expected to honour payment, and if this service is to be used the financial risk must be accepted by the budget holder. Search and rescue aircraft often have a larger interior and are less constrained in terms of maximum take-off weight – allowing more equipment or personnel to be carried longer distances.

> All requests for helicopter transfer must be made to the local ambulance service trust by a senior member of staff who can authorise payment if required.

## 17.3 Applying the ACCEPT approach to air transfers

### A – Assess (the patient and situation)

The job of the air crew is to provide facilities for transfer. They may have knowledge of advanced life support, but they should not be expected to provide expert medical or nursing care during transfer. The air ambulance service will usually arrange connecting transport with road ambulances if required. However, it is vital that this aspect of the transfer is discussed, agreed and documented to prevent unnecessary delays.

The information likely to be needed when contacting air ambulance services is:

- Name and age (date of birth) of patient
- Location of patient and planned destination
- Diagnosis
- Condition severity
- Team details (location and number)
- Equipment accompanying patient (weight may be limited)
- Requests for family or carer to accompany
- Disturbed or infectious patients must be discussed with the pilot in command at the planning stage.

## C – Control

The pilot is the team leader and is in overall charge of the aircraft and its occupants. The pilot and crew's primary responsibility is to ensure the safety of the aircraft and its occupants. Their instructions must be obeyed. It is their decision whether to undertake the transfer or even to abort a mission and land at an unplanned destination. In a helicopter air ambulance undertaking an inter-facility transfer, there may be only room for one medical attendant. If present, an air ambulance paramedic will be available to assist, but they also have a role in assisting the pilot with communications and navigation. There is generally more space available in a fixed-wing aircraft, although interventions en route remain difficult.

## C – Communication

Lines of communication should be established between those retrieving or dispatching the patient, the aircrew and the medical staff at the destination. The systematic approach to communication set out earlier in Chapter 7 lends itself to the field of aviation transfer medicine as messages, often transmitted by radio, and through third parties, need to be succinct.

Named individuals and telephone numbers should be identified and documented for liaison purposes. A central person or point of communication should be agreed where possible. Communication from aircraft is usually carried out by radio. Aircraft operational frequencies allow communication between the aircraft and civil and military airfields. In the majority of cases it will not be possible to communicate directly between the aircraft and a land-based ambulance control centre, hospital switchboard or emergency department.

> Communications are usually relayed, and must therefore be clear and concise and where possible should be through a single individual or point of contact.

Noise levels inside helicopters necessitate the use of headsets and microphones to communicate. Once on board, familiarisation with the headsets is a priority as this will be the primary method of communication during the transfer. At critical phases of flight (e.g. take-off and landing), the medical passengers and pilots will often all be 'connected'. At these times medical communication must be limited to the essentials.

During the flight, the medical passengers are often 'switched' onto a private channel where they can communicate without distracting the crew flying the aircraft. Communication is generally easier in fixed-wing aircraft due to the reduced noise levels. However, the medical team may still communicate with the flight crew via headsets. Some aircraft have satellite telephones or information can be relayed to the ground via the crew. Mobile phones should not be used on board aircraft without the express permission of the pilot.

Audible alarm systems on patient monitors are difficult or impossible to hear in a helicopter, as is escaping gas from a cylinder that has been inadvertently switched on. These alarms are also difficult to hear in a fixed-wing aircraft. It is advisable therefore to divide up visual monitoring responsibilites among the flight crew where possible.

## E – Evaluation

The potential benefits of air transfer must be weighed against the risks and limitations:

- A hostile, unfamiliar environment
- Very limited scope for medical intervention during flights
- Transfer by air may not shorten the duration of the journey if land-based vehicles must be used at each end

It may be appropriate that competent patients/parents/guardians are involved in the risk/benefit analysis so that their views can be taken into account.

> The decision to transfer by air rather than road should be given careful consideration and the rationale clearly documented.

## P – Preparation

### Patient

The patient's physiological condition should be optimised as far as possible for the transfer. Access to the patient will be difficult in the confined aircraft environment where assessment and intervention are more challenging. Most helicopter air ambulances do not fly at altitudes greater than 1500 feet (450 m). At this altitude there is little reduction in barometric pressure, although trapped air will expand and there will be a small reduction in the partial pressure of oxygen. In the pressurised cabin of a fixed-wing air ambulance there is approximately 25% less oxygen than at ground level.

Use the ABCDEF approach.

- *Airway*: Security of the airway is particularly important given the multiple patient loading/unloading episodes. Endotracheal cuffs should be inflated with water rather than air to prevent cuff distension resulting in tracheal damage, or regular assessment of cuff pressure should be undertaken

- *Breathing*: Pneumothoraces require chest drains fitted with Heimlich valves. The reduction in partial pressure of oxygen at altitude may require an increase in fractional inspired oxygen concentration

- *Circulation*: A minimum of two points of intravenous access should be secured. Consider preparing boluses of fluid and inotrope infusions in advance (these may be difficult to prepare once underway). Fluid bags that contain any air may pressurise at altitude resulting in a more rapid flow rate

- *Disability*: Intracranial air that may be present following a traumatic head injury will expand at altitude. It is recommended that these patients only travel by air in an aircraft pressurised to sea level

- *Exposure*: Ensure that patient temperature is maintained. Helicopters (especially military) can be quite cold

- *Expansion*: Remember any trapped gas will expand at altitude potentially causing pressure effects. Notably, nasogastric tubes should be kept on free drainage to deflate the stomach. 'Bi-valve' plaster casts if present

- *Family*: Ensure that the patient and their family (as appropriate) are fully consulted and briefed regarding the transfer plan

### Staff

Staff selected to undertake medical care in the air must be medically fit. An individual's propensity for motion or air sickness may influence the choice of personnel. Non-sedating prophylaxis in the form of medications such as cinnarizine can be instituted at a suitable interval prior to departure.

Although little medical intervention can be achieved in flight, constant vigilance and care is required during the transportation to and from the aircraft. This requires competent and experienced medical staff. In addition, the European Aviation Safety Agency requires that any staff assigned to travel in any aircraft must receive a briefing from the crew including the location and operation of emergency exits, the use of communication equipment, the use of specialist medical equipment and the location and use of fire extinguishers.

Staff undertaking aeromedical transport are strongly recommended to engage in initial and refresher training with the aircrew, including human factors and normal/abnormal operations.

## P – Packaging

### Patient

Packaging the patient for an air transfer requires meticulous planning. As well as adopting the ABCDEF approach as described in Chapter 9, additional thought must be given to the problems of air transport, and in particular, helicopter transfer.

Electrical equipment may emit electromagnetic radiation which could interfere with navigational or other onboard electrical systems. Any electronic medical equipment such as ventilators, monitors and syringe drivers that will be required for use in the aircraft must be approved by the Civil Aviation Authority (CAA). The approval has to specify the type and model of equipment, and the type and model of aircraft.

Most air ambulance services have some form of pre-hospital care ventilator and simple monitoring system. Inevitably there will be several stages to the journey; equipment may have to be changed at each stage. Oxygen supplies on a helicopter are limited and you cannot easily stop to pick up more.

Part of the transfer process will inevitably mean that the patient is exposed to the elements and heat loss can be a problem.

In an air ambulance, there are often a limited number of headphones that allow communication. In a helicopter, all passengers will require ear defenders of some sort. Conscious patients may find the sudden changes in noises and vibration, such as when a helicopter is about to land, frightening and this should be considered when headphones are in short supply.

Therapeutic equipment and supplies should be small and compact, easily securable and visible. All necessary drugs and equipment should be carried in an appropriately designed pack for ease of identification, preparation and use. A small case, or other stowage bag, should be taken in which to pack equipment for the return journey.

> For helicopters, head, ear and eye protection will be required for both the conscious patient and all members of the team.

### Staff

Accompanying personnel should carry the minimum personal equipment: a mobile telephone with useful telephone numbers, identification, some cash and a snack. Helicopter teams should wear protective goggles, helmets, flame retardant flight suits and appropriate footware. Ad hoc transport teams may have to improvise.

Transport back to base for personnel and equipment should be organised before the transfer is undertaken, as air ambulances are unlikely to be able to give medical teams a lift home due to the high operating costs.

> Close liason with the air ambulance provider and the aircrew at all stages is vital in helping to understand the specific preparation and packaging requirements for air transfer.

## T – Transportation

The environment inside an aircraft has some unusual features. Most air ambulance designs have overcome some of the problems, but they are still cramped. This is particularly true in a helicopter. Figure 17.1 shows an EC 135 helicopter configured for three 'passengers' and a stretcher.

The main problems can be summarised as:

- Lack of manoeuvring space
- Lack of space for supplies
- Relatively noisy – staff may need to wear headphones to communicate
- Limited number of seats

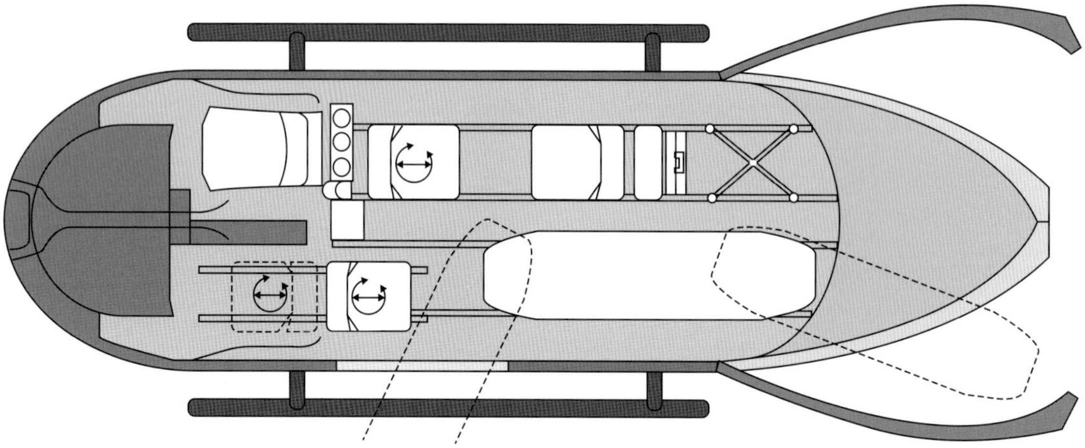

**Figure 17.1 EC 135 helicopter configured for three 'passengers' and a stretcher.** Courtesy of Bond Air Services UK

Aircraft such as the Augusta Westland 139 or 189 and Sikorsky S92 are not limited for space. However, seating may be at more than an arm's length from the patient, making access difficult. Furthermore, because the aircraft has many functions and has not been specifically designed for the transfer of patients, there may be no purpose-built anchorage points for a stretcher. In a helicopter, the noise level is high; staff can be distracted and may suffer fatigue. Vibration can be disconcerting and makes visualisation of monitor screens difficult. A few moments arranging equipment, patient and personnel with the assistance and advice of the aircrew is invaluable.

On helicopters, staff accompanying patients may be required to wear a safety helmet with built-in headphones or simply headphones. A heavy helmet makes head movement feel awkward, and the intercom sounds quiet and distant. When 'switched in' to the communications system, it is often difficult for the novice to ascertain who is talking to whom, and using the voice-operated microphone system is a skill in itself. The use of headphones and the noisy environment may render alarms on medical equipment inaudible. Equipment with visible alarm systems should be used if possible. End tidal $CO_2$ monitoring is a valuble visual confirmation of ventilation in these circumstances.

Few hospitals are equipped with a helicopter landing area immediately outside their doors. It is therefore common for patients requiring transfer by air to be taken to the aircraft by a road vehicle, and delivered to the hospital at their destination in the same way. Thus during transfer the patient will be moved to a new location several times. Each vehicle transfer represents a period of increased risk and additional transfer time for the patient. Endotracheal tubes and IV lines can be pulled out, ventilators can become disconnected and the medical team may be distracted. Care and good communication within the team is essential.

## 17.4 Retrieval of patients from helicopters

Most NHS staff will never actually transfer a patient in a helicopter; they are more likely to have to assist in the retrieval of a patient from a helicopter which has landed at their hospital. General guidelines for NHS trusts on their responsibilities for providing safety arrangements for landing helicopters are long overdue. Such guidelines should cover:

- Landing site preparation
- Retrieval team staff safety including personal protective equipment
- Approaching a helicopter

### Landing site preparation

Helicopters can only land at hospitals that have a purpose-built landing site which has been surveyed to the satisfaction of the air ambulance service operator. The hospital, or site operator, then has the responsibility to ensure that it keeps the site airworthy.

- Site operators should ensure vigilance in respect of building work, which may cause unidentified obstructions and hazards to landing aircraft
- Where possible, the site should be inspected prior to every landing to ensure that the area is clear of debris. Items such as tin cans, paper and plastic sheeting can be sucked into the aircraft engine air intake, causing catastrophic engine failure; such debris can also cause personal injury to ground retrieval team members

- Site operators should ensure that a designated assembly point is identified, and positioned at a safe distance from the actual landing point. The assembly area should be positioned such that the team can clearly see the pilot and their hand signals
- The road ambulance should be parked in a designated safe area; the vehicle should be positioned facing the aircraft in order to reduce the possibility that a down draft slams any open doors shut, trapping staff
- All non-essential personnel and spectators must be kept away from the landing area and assembly point at all times during the operation. Particular care should be taken if children or animals are in the area. Hospital security and/or police officers should be available at the site. Security vigilance must be maintained until the helicopter has left the site and is well on its way
- Fire and accidents are very rare; however, there is an increased risk of fire if the aircraft is being refuelled. Helicopter landing sites without immediate provision for fire fighting (equipment and trained personnel at the landing pad) will need to develop contingency plans with the local fire service

### Retrieval team staff safety

Personal protective equipment should be provided for, and used by, any staff who will be part of a retrieval team:

- High visibility jacket
- Eye protection – preferably anti-misting goggles to be compliant with BS166-345
- Ear defenders appropriate for the noise levels and anticipated frequencies and compliant with BS351-1
- Headgear may be considered as an optional extra, but should not interfere with the efficient fitting of ear protectors and eye protection

In addition, footwear must be robust outdoor shoes – operating theatre clogs and high heels are not appropriate. Warm trousers should be worn; female staff must not wear dresses or skirts.

### Approaching a helicopter

Only members of a ground retrieval team who have the specified personal protective equipment should be allowed to approach the helicopter. The team should position itself in an assembly area from where it can see the helicopter and vice versa. No one on the ground should approach the aircraft until the pilot (or co-pilot) makes a clear hand signal to do so. If in doubt, wait. (In general, the crew of most air ambulances will send one of its crew members away from the aircraft to meet and escort the retrieval team towards the aircraft.)

The approach should be made from the front of the aircraft keeping in full view of the pilot, initially, and, later, the crewman at the door to the aircraft. Never approach the helicopter from the rear. Tail rotor blades are lethal and may not be visible. If on a hill or sloping ground, approach and leave on the down-hill side, in order to avoid the main rotor. Remember that when stopped, the main rotor blades dip down towards the tip. If it becomes necessary to move from one side of the aircraft to the other, having previously reached the fuselage, go around the nose and within arm's length of the aircraft.

Approach a helicopter:

- Only when clearly instructed
- In clear view of the pilot

## 17.5 Fixed-wing air transfers

Most fixed-wing medical transfers are undertaken as a retrieval service by specialists; the international repatriation of sick or injured patients is a booming business. These repatriations require a great deal of forward planning, as flight slots have to be booked some time in advance. The repatriation teams often have to deal with different styles of healthcare in other countries as well as the problems of differing languages, which may lead to confusion.

When hospital staff are involved in the negotiations around the international repatriation of patients, it is important to record the following details:

- The name of the repatriation company
- The contact person's name

- Telephone number (and fax number)
- The repatriation company's patient reference number
- The patient's name
- The patient's current location

Some long distance air transfers involve the use of commercial airlines (see later in this chapter) and the need to remove up to eight seats in a potentially already overbooked flight. Aviation authorities, including the UK's CAA, usually strictly limit the carriage of any additional oxygen supplies on an aircraft.

In the developed world, fixed-wing aeromedical transfers are inter-hospital tertiary transfers, as opposed to primary and secondary missions, which are more commonly flown in helicopter air ambulances. In the UK, these transfers may be arranged for patients in relatively remote district hospitals such as the Channel Islands or Isle of Man moving to a tertiary referral centre on the mainland. More commonly, however, fixed-wing transfers involve the repatriation of patients in hospitals overseas to their local hospital in the UK.

## Planning and preparation

These missions involve complex planning and logistics, often between two or more hospitals in different countries. There may be difficulties in terms of language and culture or in obtaining up-to-date medical information from the transferring hospital. Take-off and landing slots will need to be arranged with at least two airports and ground transportation in ambulances, in different countries, will need to be carefully integrated into the overall plan and schedule for the mission.

Depending on the clinical condition of the patient, the transfer may be undertaken in a fixed-wing air ambulance or onboard a commercial airliner. Patients requiring more than general ward level care are generally transferred in an air ambulance. The level of equipment and staffing will also differ depending on whether the transfer is by air ambulance or commercial airliner.

## Fixed-wing air ambulances

A fixed-wing air ambulance is a small aircraft that has been internally modified to carry medical patients. These aircraft may be jets such as the Learjet or Citation, or may be turboprops such as the Kingair. The equipment available on these aircraft is analogous to a 'flying ICU bay', and they are staffed correspondingly, usually with a doctor and nurse experienced in intensive care and aviation medicine. There may be one or two pilots on board and potentially some space for a relative, which is at the discretion of the pilot and treating clinicians.

Although fixed-wing air ambulances offer more space and opportunity for in-flight treatments than in a helicopter air ambulance, access and space remain limited and interventions during the transfer may be difficult and dangerous. Patients must be stabilised and 'fit to fly' prior to departure.

Clearly, great care needs to be taken when planning the equipment to take on board and each piece of equipment needs to be meticulously checked prior to departure. Oxygen supplies should be carefully considered and operational redundancy built-in to all areas.

## Commercial airliner transfers

Commercial aeromedical transfers may be undertaken, in theory, in any kind of commercial airliner, operated by any airline. Each airline will have its own set of standard operating procedures and the organisers of the transfer need to liase closely with the airline to ensure a safe transfer.

An assessment of the patient's fitness to fly is important in any aeromedical transfer, but is arguably even more important when considering an airliner, both due to the relative lack of equipment available to the transferring staff and the commercial considerations of the airline.

These transfers may be staffed by a flight nurse, a flight doctor, or both, depending upon the clinical assessment of the patient. Most patients transferred by commercial airliner are at least partially ambulant due to the difficulties of getting a stretcher onboard. However, it is common to reserve a row (or more) of seats on the aircraft, both for ease of access and for patient comfort. It may not be possible (due to airline restrictions) or practical to carry loose oxygen cylinders on board and an oxygen concentrator is a common alternative. Other equipment is usually carried in a transfer bag(s) similar to those used in UK hospitals for intra-hospital transfers.

## 17.6 Common physiological considerations

A full description of all of the considerations when undertaking a fixed-wing aeromedical transfer is beyond the scope of this text, but some common issues to consider include the following.

### Hypoxia

Under normal flight conditions most air ambulances and commercial airliners have cabins pressurized to approximately 8000 feet (2400 m). At this altitude, approximately 25% less oxygen is available to breathe and patients with cardiorespiratory disease may become symptomatic below this altitude.

### Hypobaric considerations

The lower ambient pressure in the cabin in relation to sea level leads to expansion of gas-filled spaces. Any gas-containing body cavity may cause problems during the transfer, for example a simple pneumothorax may become a tension pneumothorax or gas within an obstructed bowel may lead to a perforation. Air within the cuff of an endotracheal tube will expand and consideration of replacement of the air with a liquid such as saline or sterile water should be made.

### Motion problems

Aircraft can be subject to extremes of acceleration and deceleration forces, as well as vertical shear and vibration, during periods of air turbulence. Perfusion of tissues may become compromised, especially in a hypovolaemic patient and fragile tissues may be injured. For example, unstable spinal fractures need to have special consideration, as would conditions of raised intracranial pressure.

## 17.7 Summary

The information in this chapter is presented as an introduction only. Specialist air transfer training is not covered in detail either in this manual or on the NAPSTaR course.

The safe transfer of patients by air requires an understanding of the benefits and limitations of this mode of transfer. Helicopter landings need to be undertaken under controlled conditions and safety is a paramount consideration. Understanding some of the problems of the international repatriation of patients may help receiving hospitals.

# CHAPTER 18
# Respiratory support and the patient with a difficult airway or tracheostomy

## Learning outcomes

After reading this chapter, you will be able to:
- Describe how and when to transport unintubated patients
- Assess patients with potentially difficult airways and know how they may be managed
- Describe how to transfer a patient with a tracheostomy
- Recognise a blocked tracheostomy
- Recognise oxygen supplies and fittings
- Calculate oxygen supply requirement

## 18.1 Introduction

The airway of the patient should be considered carefully during the initial assessment phase of the transfer.

For the intubated patient, the size of tube should be checked and its position confirmed by chest X-ray. It should be well secured and the patient adequately sedated and paralysed to prevent tube movement during transfer.

For the non-intubated patient, if there is doubt regarding the security of the airway or adequacy of ventilation, the safest option will usually be to intubate the patient prior to transfer. A possible difficult airway is likely to be even more difficult to manage in an isolated environment en route. Emergency airway management outside the operating theatre is known to be associated with more frequent problems than routine anaesthesia. The consultant in charge of the transfer is responsible for considering these risks and selecting a team with the appropriate skills, equipment and training to manage any potential deterioration.

There may be occasions when the risks of attempting to secure an unstable airway outweigh that of attempting to transfer the patient unintubated, possibly due to a need for specialist skills or equipment not available at the transferring unit. These transfers can be extremely challenging and require the most senior team available.

When transferring an unintubated patient, any compromise with their airway or breathing is likely to worsen if they become upset or agitated.

An accompanying parent is likely to be the best person to keep a young patient calm. In these circumstances the parent effectively becomes a part of the transfer team and they should be briefed both on what to expect and what is expected of them. It should be agreed in advance that the parent will vacate the immediate clinical area should a crisis occur. In an ambulance this might be achieved by sitting in the cab with the driver/paramedic whilst the vehicle is parked up and the situation resolved.

*Neonatal, Adult and Paediatric Safe Transfer and Retrieval: A Practical Approach to Transfers*, First Edition.
Edited by Bernard Foëx, Peter-Marc Fortune and Cassie Lawn.
© 2019 John Wiley & Sons Ltd. Published 2019 by John Wiley & Sons Ltd.

## 18.2 Respiratory support – applying oxygen

### Oxygen cylinders

It is important to have a basic understanding of oxygen supplies. Most oxygen cylinders are made of steel; however, there is trend away from this traditional material towards 'hood-wrapped' advanced steel carbon fibre (aramid), better known by trade names such as Kevlar®. This is also used in bullet-proof vests and aircraft body parts, for example.

Steel cylinders are graded by size, the commonest ones used in NHS wards and departments are D, E and F sizes (Table 18.1). All UK steel oxygen cylinders are filled to a pressure of 137 bars (1 bar = 1 atmos = 14.7 psi = 101.33 kPa). Lightweight carbon fibre cylinders are filled to a higher pressure.

**Table 18.1** Oxygen cylinder characteristics

|  | D | E | F |
|---|---|---|---|
| Common usage | Portable | Anaesthetic 'machines' | Emergency department trolleys Theatre trolleys |
| Capacity (litres) | 340 | 680 | 1360 |
| Connection | Pin-index | Pin-index | Bull-nosed |

For a given temperature there is a linear relationship between the pressure ($P$) in the cylinder and the volume ($V$) of the gas (Boyle's law: $P_1 \times V_1 = P_2 \times V_2$); therefore, as the contents of the cylinder reduce so does the pressure on the gauge. A full E-sized cylinder will contain 680 litres of gas; when the gauge reads half full, the cylinder will contain 340 litres.

If an oxygen flowmeter is set to deliver 10 l/min, a full E-sized cylinder will be empty in 68 minutes (680/10), and a half filled E-sized cylinder will be empty in 34 minutes, after which time there will be no gas or pressure left in the cylinder.

### Connections and keys

It is important to understand the component parts of the connections between a gas cylinder and the oxygen delivery system. The pressure in compressed gas cylinders must be reduced before it reaches a flowmeter or ventilator. This reduction in pressure is accomplished using a regulator. The connection to the regulator may be either a pin-index system or a bull-nosed fitting (Table 18.1, Figures 18.1 and 18.2).

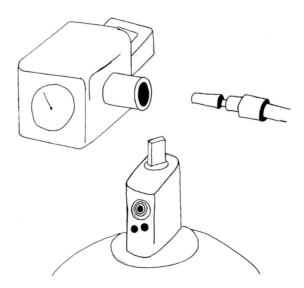

**Figure 18.1 Pin-index fittings**

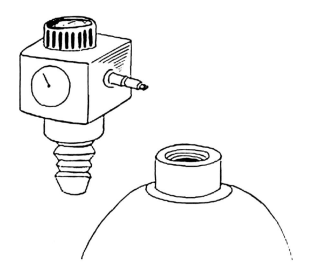

**Figure 18.2 Bull-nosed fittings**

In the UK, all D- and E-sized oxygen cylinders have a pin-index fitting system. The pin-index system is specific to the medical gas to be supplied, and ensures only the correct gas can be connected to the regulator. Larger cylinders, F-sized and above, do not have this gas-specific anti-error device. Cylinders containing other medical gases, such as medical air, could potentially be connected to the regulator.

Oxygen regulators have either a flowmeter/nipple for direct connection to oxygen mask tubing or a resuscitation circuit as described later in this chapter, or a Schrader socket which connects to a white pressure hose leading to a ventilator. Like the pin-index fitting, the Schrader probe and collar index system is unique to medical gas. Newer lightweight cylinders have a built-in combination regulator with both Schrader socket and nipple outlets. In the event of a ventilator failure, you can attach and use a resuscitation circuit without the need for a second cylinder with the appropriate connections.

In order to plan the requirement for oxygen supplies during a journey, a working knowledge of oxygen masks, breathing circuits and ventilators is necessary.

## Oxygen delivery systems in the spontaneously breathing patient

Oxygen masks are part of everyday life in UK hospitals, although the theory of their operation is often poorly understood by those who use them. The amount of oxygen delivered may vary with the patient's respiratory effort. Oxygen masks are rarely used in neonatal patients.

### Variable performance oxygen devices

The oxygen mask most frequently seen in hospitals is the Hudson type (Figure 18.3). This clear plastic mask with an oxygen nipple and side holes is designed to deliver up to 50% oxygen in most patients. The normal inspiratory flow pattern is sinusoidal. The inspiratory:expiratory time ratio varies from 1:1 to 1:2, and the peak inspiratory flow rate is approximately 3–4 times the minute volume (i.e. 20–30 l/min at rest). The peak inspiratory flow rate is related to the tidal volume.

During the first second of inspiration, the patient initially breathes the oxygen mixture from inside the mask. Then air will be entrained through the holes in the mask, thus diluting the total inhaled oxygen mixture. If the patient takes a deeper breath they will entrain more air, and thus the inspired oxygen concentration will fall. So, the concentration of inhaled oxygen varies with the tidal volume or peak inspiratory flow rate. Such masks are therefore classified as *variable performance masks*. The instruction leaflet that indicates the percentage oxygen at varying flow rates is, therefore, only an approximation (Table 18.2).

During expiration, much of the expired gas, containing $CO_2$, passes out through the holes, preventing the accumulation of $CO_2$, so-called 'rebreathing'. The residual expired breath in the mask is flushed out by the continuous flow of oxygen during the pause between expiration and inspiration. Thus the amount of rebreathing is affected by the oxygen flow and the size of the mask – the reservoir. Larger masks and very low flows of oxygen (less than 5 l/min) would encourage rebreathing.

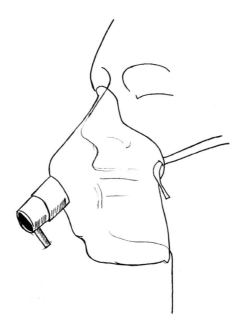

**Figure 18.3 Oxygen mask – Hudson type (side holes not shown)**

| Table 18.2 Percentage oxygen at varying flow rates – Hudson mask (approximate) | |
| --- | --- |
| **Oxygen flow rate (l/min)** | **Oxygen concentration (%)** |
| 5 | 35 |
| 6 | 40 |
| 8 | 50 |

Dual prong nasal cannulae or 'nasal specs' perform like a variable performance mask. The gas reservoir, instead of being the empty space inside the mask, is the volume of the nasopharynx. Breathing in with the mouth closed will allow oxygen flow and some air entrainment through the nose. Breathing in with the mouth open would allow more air entrainment and dilute the inspired concentration of oxygen. The quoted inspired oxygen levels for nasal cannulae are of the same order as variable performance masks (Table 18.3).

| Table 18.3 Percentage oxygen at varying flow rates in nasal cannulae | |
| --- | --- |
| **Oxygen flow rate (l/min)** | **Oxygen concentration (%)** |
| 1 | 24 |
| 2 | 27 |
| 3 | 30 |
| 4 | 33 |
| 5 | 36 |
| 6 | 42 |

The formula for the inspired concentration of oxygen with nasal specs is 21% + (3 × oxygen flow rate (l/min)). Neonates can generally tolerate a maximum of 1 l/min.

Flows higher than 6 l/min are not well tolerated, and dry out the mucous membranes. In neonates flows of >0.5 l/min are likely to cause nasal irritation. These masks are not used in neonatal patients.

The efficiency of variable performance oxygen masks and nasal cannulae depends on the tidal volume and the size of the reservoir. Masks are useful in patients who are strictly mouth breathers as well as some patients with extreme nasal irritation or epistaxis. On the negative side, masks are uncomfortable and confining, muffle communication and they interfere with eating. Nasal cannulae are generally much better tolerated in children and mildly confused patients; however, they should be correctly fitted and supervised.

Increasing the size of the reservoir and filling it with an oxygen mixture may overcome the problem of air entrainment. Non-rebreathing masks are fitted with a reservoir bag and a one-way valve to prevent mixing of expired gas with the reservoir gas. Oxygen flows into the reservoir bag at 8–10 l/min. When the patient breathes in, the gas mixture from the mask is inhaled first, followed by gas from the reservoir bag. Providing the reservoir bag is filled before use, and the mask is close fitting, there should be no air entrainment. Expired air containing $CO_2$ is vented through one-way valves built into the mask. Such devices are capable of delivering up to 90% oxygen (Figure 18.4).

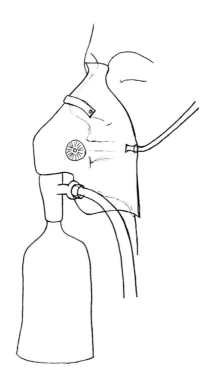

**Figure 18.4  Oxygen mask with reservoir**

## Fixed performance masks

In some cases it is important to control the percentage of inspired oxygen accurately despite variations in tidal volume and peak inspiratory flow rates. This is achieved using a *fixed performance* oxygen-driven Venturi mask to ensure that the gas mixture is supplied at a rate which is guaranteed to be higher than the peak inspiratory flow (Figure 18.5). These masks are not used in neonatal patients.

The design of the Venturi system is such that a constant proportion of air is entrained when the oxygen flow exceeds a certain minimal level. Since a total gas flow rate of 40 l/min is usually adequate to satisfy the peak inspiratory flow rate of the patient, the concentration of oxygen is controlled by using different entrainment ratios for each oxygen concentration. The instructions with each 24%, 28%, 40% or 60% oxygen mask tell the user what flow rate of oxygen to put into the mask to achieve the desired concentration of oxygen inside the mask. Table 18.4 gives approximate values.

Such a mask provides a micro-environment around the face. This makes the exact positioning of the mask less critical and keeps the patient's face cool. The high flow rate effectively eliminates rebreathing and ensures that only pre-mixed gas is inhaled. These masks are not used in neonatal patients.

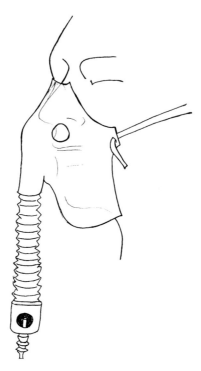

**Figure 18.5 Fixed performance mask – Venturi type**

| Table 18.4 Typical entrainment ratios used to provide different oxygen concentrations in Venturi masks | | | | |
|---|---|---|---|---|
| Oxygen flow (l/min) | Air entrained (l/min) | Ratio (air:$O_2$) | Oxygen concentration (%) | Total flow (l/min) |
| 2 | 51 | 25:1 | 24 | 53 |
| 4 | 41 | 10:1 | 28 | 45 |
| 8 | 25 | 3:1 | 40 | 33 |
| 12 | 20 | 5:3 | 50 | 32 |
| 15 | 15 | 1:1 | 60 | 30 |

## 18.3 Calculating oxygen supplies

A simple oxygen consumption calculation should be made when planning the transportation of a patient. First, ascertain what flow rate of oxygen is required to deliver the desired percentage of oxygen, whether this is done using a mask, a resuscitation circuit or a ventilator. Then total the journey time and its component parts. The journey to the ambulance, the ambulance journey and the journey from the ambulance at the other end will each contribute to the total oxygen consumption, although different cylinders may be used.

It is important to plan for the worst case scenario such as a major delay at any stage or a mechanical failure of the ventilator. It is a useful rule of thumb to provide oxygen for twice the anticipated journey time.

## 18.4 Spontaneous breathing and resuscitation circuits

**The highest oxygen consumption by an oxygen mask or adult breathing circuit is 15 l/min.**

### Self-inflating resuscitation bag with one-way valve

The self-inflating resuscitation circuit is commonly referred to as bag–valve–mask or an Ambu bag. The system enables the operator to manually inflate the lungs via a tight fitting face mask to create a seal. The bag is made of silicone rubber, which, after squeezing, will re-expand due to its own elasticity. This means that the device can be used to manually inflate the lungs even in the absence of an oxygen supply. In most cases there is a second reservoir bag attached to the silicone bag (Figure 18.6). If attached to an oxygen supply, during spontaneous respiration the patient may inspire an oxygen enriched gas mixture from the silicone bag. With the reservoir attached, it is possible to reach inspired oxygen concentrations of 90%. In the event of oxygen failure, the patient can entrain air via a built-in valve. Due to the resistance of the valves in the system, a bag–valve–mask is not suitable for delivering oxygen to small, spontaneously breathing children.

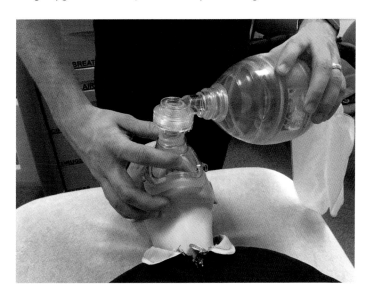

**Figure 18.6 Bag–valve–mask.** Courtesy of Paul Reavley

As they are not always single-patient-use items the bag–valve–mask and anaesthetic circuits below should always be used with a bacterial filter placed between the circuit and the face mask.

> **The self-inflating resuscitation circuit with one-way valve and filter should be considered as a mandatory piece of transfer equipment for all circumstances.**

## Anaesthetic circuits

These circuits require specific training for their proper use and must not be used by the untrained. It is also vital to note that failure of the oxygen supply renders these circuits useless.

### Mapleson C (Waters) breathing circuit

In adults and older children (>25 kg) a breathing circuit favoured by anaesthetists is the Mapleson C or Waters circuit (Figure 18.7). The system is designed to be attached to a tight fitting anaesthetic face mask which is held in place over the patient's nose and mouth by the operator to create a seal. Oxygen is fed into the system between the reservoir bag and the spill valve, providing a large reservoir from which the patient can breathe. However, during expiration the expired gas containing $CO_2$ is mixed in the reservoir bag with incoming oxygen. As the bag distends, excess pressure is vented through an adjustable spill valve. There is great potential for rebreathing and accumulation of $CO_2$ because unlike the non-rebreathing masks described earlier, there is no one-way valve between the mask and the reservoir. Increasing the oxygen flow rate to at least three times the patient's minute volume, or 15 l/min in adults, will flush the reservoir and minimise rebreathing.

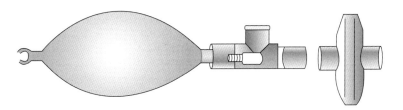

**Figure 18.7 The Mapleson C circuit**

The Mapleson C circuit allows the delivery of 100% oxygen and may be used to manually inflate the lungs by squeezing the reservoir bag, but only in the presence of an oxygen supply.

### Mapleson F breathing circuit (Ayre's T-piece)

This breathing circuit is favoured by intensivists and anaesthetists in small children because it presents virtually no resistance to expiration, is able to deliver positive end expiratory pressure (PEEP) and it provides tactile feedback on the status of the child's lungs. The system is designed to be attached to a close fitting face mask that is held in place over the child's nose and mouth to create a seal. The oxygen supply attaches between the mask and a corrugated tube with an open ended bag which acts as a reservoir (Figure 18.8). This reservoir fills with a mixture of exhaled and fresh gas during expiration and fresh gas during the expiratory pause. In order to prevent rebreathing the fresh gas, flow in a spontaneously breathing child must be maintained at 2.5–3 times the child's minute volume to flush the reservoir of exhaled gas. The limited size of the reservoir means it is only suitable for children up to about 25 kg, above which a Mapleson C breathing circuit should be used.

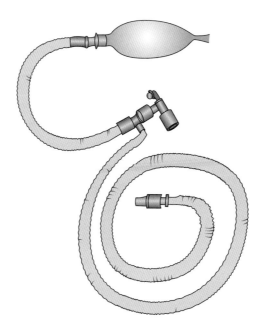

**Figure 18.8 Mapleson F circuit (Ayre's T-piece)**

## 18.5 The patient with a difficult airway

The difficult airway is defined as the clinical situation in which a conventionally trained anaesthetist experiences difficulties with face mask ventilation, tracheal intubation, or both.

These difficulties may be either expected or unexpected events. Poor airway assessment, poor planning after identifying a potentially difficult airway and not planning for failure are all identified as contributing to poor outcomes.

### Airway assessment

An airway assessment should be performed prior to anaesthesia in an attempt to identify any factors that may pose difficulties with face mask ventilation, laryngoscopy or intubation.

There is no one test that will reliably predict a difficult airway. An unexpected difficult intubation occurs in approximately 3% of adult elective anaesthetic practice, although it is thought to be less common in paediatric practice.

#### *History*

A history of previous difficulties should be an alert to potential problems, as should the existence of conditions known to be associated with a difficult airway. These may be acute conditions of the upper airway or chronic conditions with reduced joint mobility such as ankylosing spondylitis, or syndromes such as Pierre Robin and inherited lysosomal storage diseases.

## Examination

General assessment of body habitus and obvious external head and neck pathology should be carried out. Poor mouth opening, protruding or loose teeth, large tongue, small mandible and poor neck mobility can all increase difficulties.

Specific airways tests such as the modified Mallampati score (Figure 18.9) or thyromental distance can be used in isolation or as part of a multivariate scoring system. Most airway tests have not been validated for paediatric patients and may be of limited use in an uncooperative patient.

The risk of aspiration must also be assessed when planning airway management. High residual gastric volume may be drained by a nasogastric tube if in place. Rapid sequence induction with cricoid pressure aims to achieve early intubation and minimise the risk of airways contamination prior to placement of a tube in the trachea.

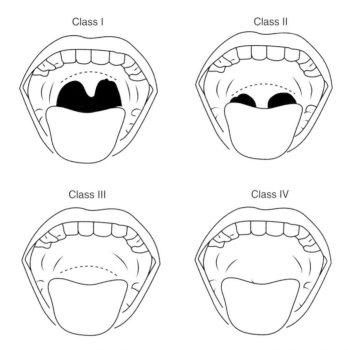

Class I      Class II      Class III      Class IV

**Figure 18.9 Modified Mallampati score, assessed by viewing the posterior pharynx with the patient sitting, looking straight ahead with the mouth wide open. Class III or IV are associated with increased difficulty in mask ventilation and laryngoscopy.**
Source: Samsoon GL, Young JR (1987) Difficult tracheal intubation: a retrospective study. *Anaesthesia* 42: 487–90. Reproduced with permission of John Wiley & Sons

## The recognised difficult airway

If airway management is identified as a potential difficulty following appropriate assessment, a strategy is required. This should be a logical sequence of plans that aim to achieve good gas exchange and prevention of aspiration whilst the airway of secured.

The plan will depend on the problem identified, the patient and the skills of the team managing the case. This may be an initial attempt at direct laryngoscopy, the use of video laryngoscopy or awake fibreoptic intubation. Increasingly, high flow nasal oxygenation is being used in such cases to allow apnoeic oxygenation and to prevent desaturation whilst the airway is secured.

In the patient with a predicted difficult airway, inhalational induction and maintenance of spontaneous ventilation is more frequently employed whilst securing the airway. For upper airway obstruction, such as croup or epiglottitis, direct laryngoscopy can be attempted to try to pass a tube through the narrowed glottis or subglottis. In patients where the laryngoscopy is likely to be problematic, video laryngoscopy or asleep fibreoptic intubation through a supraglottic airway device can be used.

If significant difficulty is anticipated, the assistance of an ENT surgeon should be sought, if possible, prior to induction of anaesthesia. Should face mask ventilation and intubation prove impossible there may be a need for an emergency surgical airway.

## The unexpected difficult airway

In the event that airway management is unexpectedly difficult, the response should be structured and practiced. The Difficult Airway Society (DAS) has published guidelines for the management of unanticipated difficult intubation, which many have now adopted. Separate guidelines exist for paediatric difficult intubation and obstetric patients (Figure 18.10).

Further details and guidelines for children aged 1–8 years can be found at www.das.uk.com.

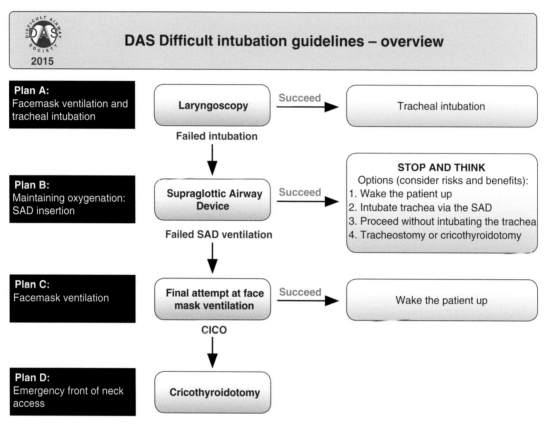

This flowchart forms part of the DAS guidelines for unanticipated difficult intubation in adults 2015 and should be used in conjunction with the text.

**Figure 18.10 Management of unanticipated difficult tracheal intubation in adults.** Source: Reproduced from Frerk C, Mitchell VS, McNarry AF, et al. (2015) Difficult Airway Society 2015 guidelines for management of unanticipated difficult intubation in adults. *Br J Anaesthesia* 115(6): 827–48. doi:10.1093/bja/aev371. Reproduced with permission of Difficult Airway Society

Plan A aims for successful face mask ventilation and tracheal intubation, with the priority being maintenance of oxygenation and anaesthesia whilst this is achieved. The likelihood of success is increased by optimal patient positioning, use of pre-oxygenation and adequate neuromuscular blockade. Techniques such as external laryngeal manipulation and the use of bougies or stylets may be helpful in achieving success. In the child, insertion of a nasogastric or orogastric tube may help manage gastric distension. The number of attempts at direct or video laryngoscopy is limited to prevent airway trauma.

If unsuccessful, a failed intubation should be declared and Plan B implemented.

Plan B focuses on insertion of a supraglottic airway device (SAD) and maintaining oxygenation and ventilation. Once achieved, a decision can be made whether to wake the patient, continue with the SAD alone, use the SAD as a conduit for intubation, or move to a surgical airway.

If oxygenation through a SAD cannot be achieved after a maximum of three attempts, failed SAD ventilation should be declared and Plan C should follow on directly.

Plan C is a final attempt at face mask ventilation to achieve oxygenation. If this is not possible, ensure full paralysis and attempt a two-person technique and use airways adjuncts. Failure is now a 'can't intubate, can't oxygenate' (CICO) situation necessitating Plan D.

Plan D is emergency front-of-neck access. In the adult population, DAS advocate a scalpel cricothyroidotomy using a scalpel, bougie and cuffed tube. There is debate regarding the optimal technique in children as the cricoid membrane is difficult to feel in the under 5 s and needle techniques are recognised to have high failure rates, even in adults.

The APLS recommend that in an emergency 'cannot intubate, cannot ventilate' situation, children up to 1 year of age should have an emergency tracheostomy, with direct visualisation of the tracheal wall. Between the ages of 1 and 5 years an emergency tracheostomy should also be used, but a cricothyroidotomy may be performed if the cricothyroid membrane can be identified. In older children and adolescents a surgical cricothyroidotomy is advised, as for adults. An ENT surgeon is likely to be the most appropriate team member to attempt a surgical airway so should be involved in the management of the difficult airway early if possible.

## 18.6 The patient with a tracheostomy

Patients with a tracheostomy should be cared for and transferred by staff appropriately trained and competent in tracheostomy care. Failure to correctly insert, securely position or appropriately care for the airway device may lead to a displaced or blocked tube, which may be fatal (Figure 18.11).

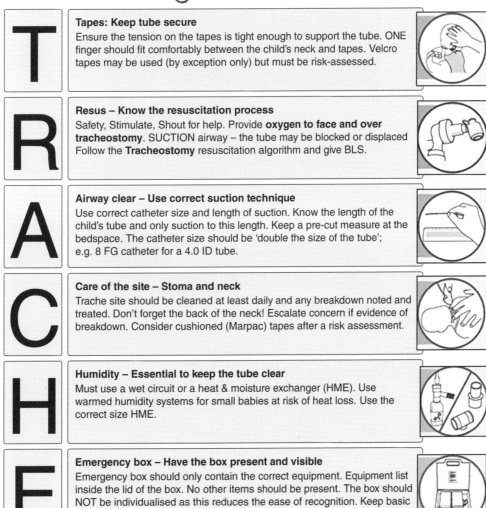

**Figure 18.11 Tracheostomy care.** Reproduced with permission of Joanne Cooke, Great Ormond Street Hospital

Emergency equipment including suction, appropriate size suction catheters, replacement tracheostomy tubes, scissors, lubricating jelly and tapes must remain with the patient at the bedside and throughout any transfer process. A heat and moisture exchanger (HME) or alternative form of humidification should be used if active humidification is discontinued. Additional resuscitation equipment may be required for individual patients or in the hospital environment.

This equipment should include the following items and should be checked daily:

- Usual size tracheostomy tube with tapes attached
- Half size smaller tracheostomy tube with tapes attached
- Suction catheter size indicated on the bedhead information
- In hospital: resuscitation trolley with self-inflating bag and face masks, two sources of oxygen, simple airway adjuncts such as oropharyngeal airways, nasopharyngeal airways and laryngeal mask airways
- Scissors
- Spare tape
- Gauze swab
- Gloves

Often all this equipment will be kept together in a specifically designed, easily identifiable case with an attached contents checklist (Figures 18.12 and 18.13).

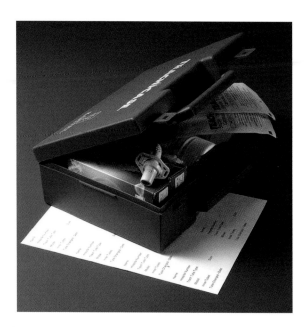

**Figure 18.12 Trachicase.** Courtesy of Kapitex Healthcare

**Tracheostomy box list**

**2 x** spare tracheostomy tubes of **same size** in a sealed package/container

Trache name and size_____ Distal length_____mm

**1 x** spare tracheostomy of **size smaller** (can be a Shiley) left in sealed package/container

Spare trache name and size_____ Distal length_____mm

| | |
|---|---|
| Cotton tapes or Collar with tapes | Lubricant gel sachet x 2 |
| Small face mask (blue) | HME appropriate for patient |
| Round ended scissors | 0.9% sodium chloride vials x 2 |
| | 2 ml syringes x 2 |

| |
|---|
| *If cuffed tracheostomy:* |
| *5 ml syringe x 1* |
| *Water vial (if balloon inflated with water)* |

**Store at head of bed:**
Additional equipment – local safety checklist (PICU airway bag / Going out bag / Community)
Oxygen
Guedel airway
High flow oxygen delivery face mask with reservoir
Self-inflating bag valve mask with oxygen reservoir and tubing
Suction and suction catheters
PPE: Gloves, Apron, Eye protection
Water for cleaning suction tubing

Tracheostomy Group V1.4 updated 09/10/2018

**Figure 18.13 Example of a tracheostomy box list.** Courtesy of Richard Neal

## Managing tracheostomy emergencies

The National Tracheostomy Safety Project paediatric guidance has received the support of the Royal College of Paediatrics and Child Health (RCPCH) and other national professional bodies: Association of Anaesthetists of Great Britain and Ireland, British Association of Prosthetists and Orthotists, Paediatric Intensive Care Society and Advanced Life Support Group. The Paediatric Working Group developed an emergency resuscitation algorithm, teaching material, bedhead signs and standardised emergency tracheostomy equipment, for use by health professionals caring for any paediatric patient with a tracheostomy. The information is available for download from www.tracheostomy.org.uk and examples are shown in Figures 18.14 and 18.15. This training package is designed for use by healthcare professionals in tertiary, non-tertiary and community environments and also by patient carers. An A6 copy of the algorithm and bedhead version is inside the tracheostomy box for use in any environment.

The aim has been to improve patient safety following reports revealing potentially avoidable harm in tracheostomy-related emergencies. The bedhead sign is designed to be displayed at the patient's bedside and contains vital airway information and the emergency resuscitation algorithm. We have an increasing number of complex patients with tracheostomies and a national increase in demand for long term ventilation and the aim is to keep this high risk population safe.

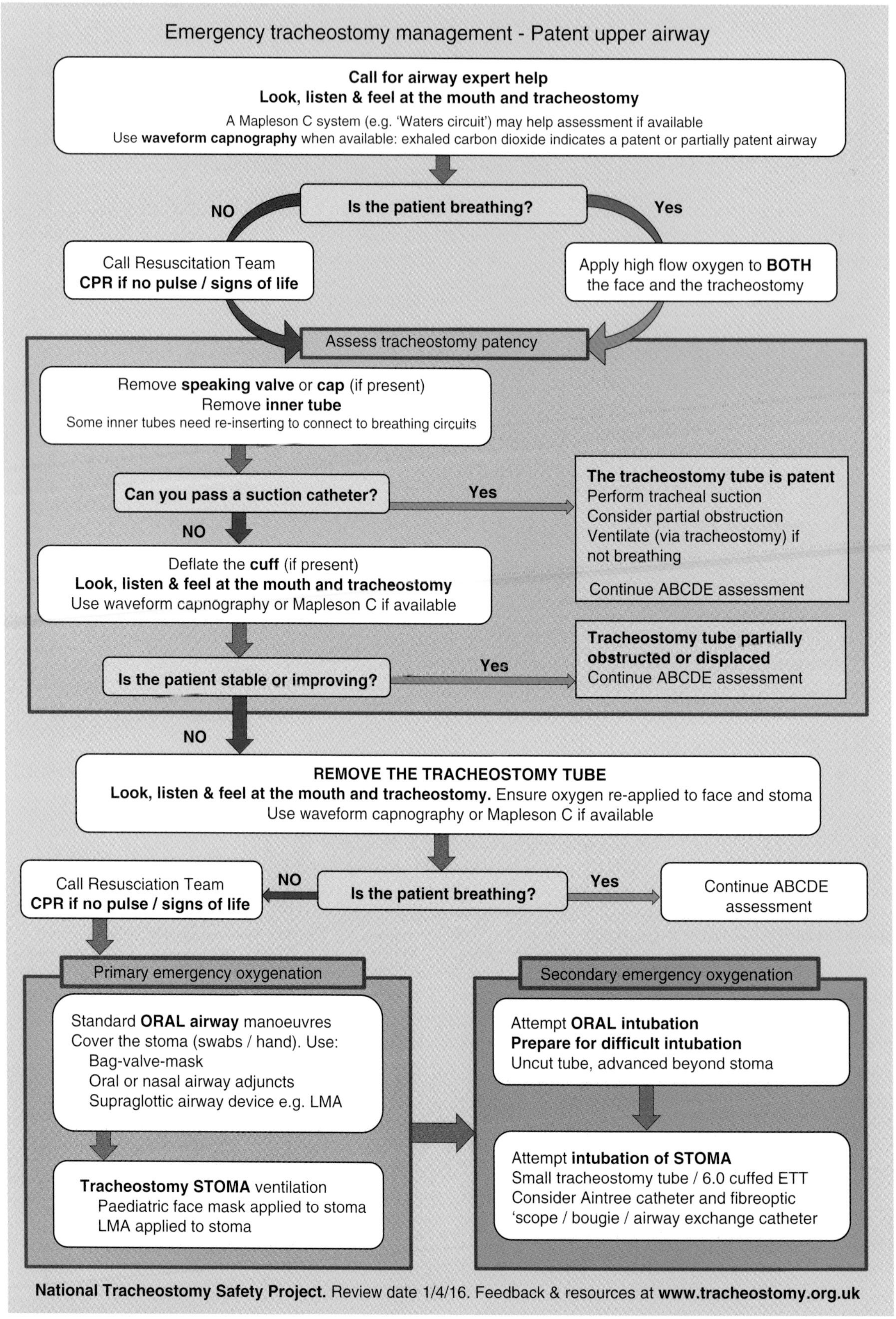

## Emergency tracheostomy management - Patent upper airway

**Call for airway expert help**
**Look, listen & feel at the mouth and tracheostomy**
A Mapleson C system (e.g. 'Waters circuit') may help assessment if available
Use **waveform capnography** when available: exhaled carbon dioxide indicates a patent or partially patent airway

**Is the patient breathing?**

NO → Call Resuscitation Team
**CPR if no pulse / signs of life**

Yes → Apply high flow oxygen to **BOTH** the face and the tracheostomy

**Assess tracheostomy patency**

Remove **speaking valve** or **cap** (if present)
Remove **inner tube**
Some inner tubes need re-inserting to connect to breathing circuits

**Can you pass a suction catheter?**

Yes → **The tracheostomy tube is patent**
Perform tracheal suction
Consider partial obstruction
Ventilate (via tracheostomy) if not breathing

Continue ABCDE assessment

NO → Deflate the **cuff** (if present)
**Look, listen & feel at the mouth and tracheostomy**
Use waveform capnography or Mapleson C if available

**Is the patient stable or improving?**

Yes → **Tracheostomy tube partially obstructed or displaced**
Continue ABCDE assessment

NO → **REMOVE THE TRACHEOSTOMY TUBE**
**Look, listen & feel at the mouth and tracheostomy.** Ensure oxygen re-applied to face and stoma
Use waveform capnography or Mapleson C if available

**Is the patient breathing?**

NO → Call Resuscitation Team
**CPR if no pulse / signs of life**

Yes → Continue ABCDE assessment

**Primary emergency oxygenation**

Standard **ORAL airway** manoeuvres
Cover the stoma (swabs / hand). Use:
  Bag-valve-mask
  Oral or nasal airway adjuncts
  Supraglottic airway device e.g. LMA

**Tracheostomy STOMA** ventilation
  Paediatric face mask applied to stoma
  LMA applied to stoma

**Secondary emergency oxygenation**

Attempt **ORAL intubation**
**Prepare for difficult intubation**
Uncut tube, advanced beyond stoma

Attempt **intubation of STOMA**
Small tracheostomy tube / 6.0 cuffed ETT
Consider Aintree catheter and fibreoptic 'scope / bougie / airway exchange catheter

**National Tracheostomy Safety Project.** Review date 1/4/16. Feedback & resources at **www.tracheostomy.org.uk**

**Figure 18.14 Emergency tracheostomy management – patent upper airway.** Source: http://www.tracheostomy.org.uk/storage/files/Patent%20Airway%20Algorithm.pdf. Reproduced with permission of National Tracheostomy Safety Project

(a)

> # This patient has a
> # New TRACHEOSTOMY
>
> **Patient ID:**    *Patient Label / Details*
>
> **Tracheostomy:**    *Add tube specification including cuff or inner tube*
>
> _____mm ID, _____mm distal length
>
> **Suction:**    _____ FG Catheter to Depth _____ cm 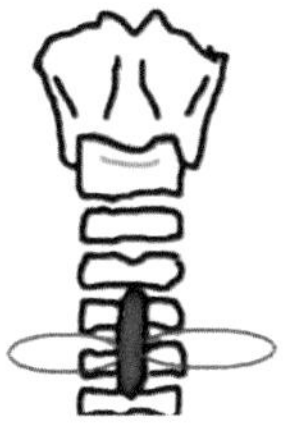
>
> **Indicate on this diagram any sutures in place**
>
> ## UPPER AIRWAY ABNORMALITY: Yes / No
> Document laryngoscopy grade and notes on upper airway management or patient specific resuscitation plans
>
> Due 1$^{st}$ tracheostomy change: ____ / ____ / ____    (by ENT ONLY)
>
> **In an Emergency: Call 2222 and request the Resuscitation Team and ENT surgeon**
> **Follow the Emergency PaediatricTracheostomy Management Algorithm on reverse**

**Figure 18.15 Examples of tracheostomy bedheads and treatment algorithm: (a) new tracheostomy bedhead, (b) tracheostomy bedhead, and (c) emergency paediatric tracheostomy management algorithm.**
Source: http://www.tracheostomy.org.uk/storage/files/NTSP%20Bedhead%20and%20Algorithm%202015_1_.pdf.
Reproduced with permission of National Tracheostomy Safety Project

(b)

| | |
|---|---|
| | This patient has a<br><br>**TRACHEOSTOMY** |

**Patient ID :** *Patient Details*

**Tracheostomy:** Add tube specification including cuff or inner tube

_____mm ID, _____ mm distal length

**Suction:** _____ FG Catheter to Depth _____ cm

**UPPER AIRWAY ABNORMALITY: Yes / No**  please give details of any expected difficulty

### Emergency Paediatric Tracheostomy Management

**SAFETY - STIMULATE - SHOUT FOR HELP - OXYGEN**

**SAFE:** Check Safe area, Stimulate, and Shout for help, CALL 2222 (hospital) or 999 (home)
**AIRWAY:** Open child's airway: head tilt / chin lift / pillow or towel under shoulders may help
**OXYGEN:** Ensure **high flow oxygen** to the **tracheostomy AND the face** as soon as oxygen available
**Capnograph:** Exhaled carbon dioxide waveform may indicate a patent airway (secondary responders)

**SUCTION TO ASSESS TRACHEOSTOMY PATENCY**

**Remove any attachments: humidifier (HME), speaking valve and change inner tube (if present)**
Inner tubes need re-inserting to connect to bagging circuits

**The tracheostomy tube is patent**
Perform tracheal suction
Consider partial obstruction
Consider tracheostomy tube change

**CONTINUE ASSESSMENT (ABCDE)**

**Can you pass a SUCTION catheter?**  Yes

No

**EMERGENCY TRACHEOSTOMY TUBE CHANGE**

Deflate cuff (if present). Reassess patency after any tube change
1st – same size tube, 2nd – smaller size tube
* 3rd – smaller size tube sited over suction catheter to guide
**IF UNSUCCESSFUL – REMOVE THE TUBE**

**IS THE PATIENT BREATHING? – Look, listen and feel at the mouth and tracheostomy/stoma**

No  Yes

**5 RESCUE BREATHS – USE TRACHEOSTOMY IF PATENT**

Patent Upper Airway – deliver breath to the mouth
Obstructed Upper Airway – deliver breath to tracheostomy/stoma

**RESPONDS:** continue oxygen, reassessment and stabilisation

Plan for definitive airway if tube change failure

**CHECK FOR SIGNS OF LIFE ? – START CPR**

15 compressions : 2 rescue breaths
Ensure help or resuscitation team called

**Basic Response**

*3-smaller size tube sited over suction catheter to guide: to be used if out of hospital

**Figure 18.15 (Continued)**

(c)

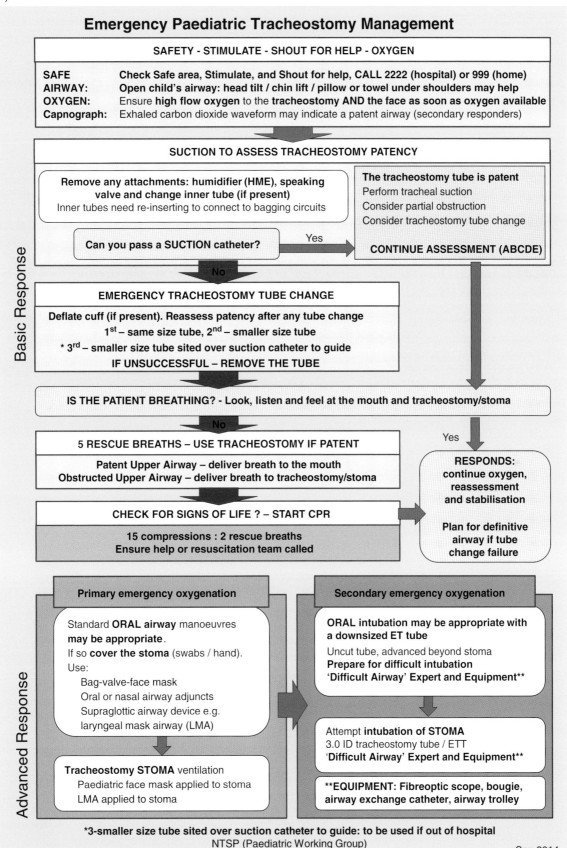

**Figure 18.15 (Continued)**

## Management of a blocked tracheostomy

When you suspect a patient with a tracheostomy tube is not breathing adequately the procedure to follow is:

- Use bedhead information regarding the patient's tracheostomy
- Use the emergency algorithm either at the bed or in the patient's tracheostomy box

***Many patients will get better by just removing the blocked tube allowing them to breathe through the stoma, or by replacing the blocked tube with a new one.***

### Basic life support

1. Stimulate the patient
2. Shout for help
3. Open and check the airway, with a head tilt/chin lift. *This exposes the tracheostomy tube* and importantly opens the upper airway
4. Apply oxygen to the face and tracheostomy when available
5. Assess the patency of the tracheostomy. This can be done by an advanced responder using a suction catheter and capnography. ***If you are unable to pass the suction catheter down the tracheostomy tube to the length on the bedhead information – then the tube must be changed immediately with the same size tube.*** If this fails to relieve the obstruction or you cannot insert it:
   - Try a size smaller tube (ideally 0.5 mm smaller or 1 mm smaller if 0.5 mm smaller tube is not available)
   - If unable to insert this, thread a suction catheter through the smaller tracheostomy tube. Insert the tip of the suction catheter into the stoma, then attempt to guide the tracheostomy tube along the catheter and into the stoma
   - If this is unsuccessful then remove the tracheostomy tube and position the neck with the stoma open
6. Check for breathing. Place the side of your face over the tracheostomy tube or face to listen and feel for any breaths, and at the same time look at the patient's chest to observe any breathing movement. If the patient is breathing satisfactorily, place them in the recovery position and continue to assess. If the patient is not breathing, or there are only infrequent gasps, you will have to give rescue breaths
7. Give five rescue breaths.
   - If you have succeeded in removing the obstructed tracheostomy and replaced it with a patent tracheostomy tube you should cover the patient's tracheostomy tube with your mouth and exhale to make the chest rise. Remove your mouth from the patient's tube to let the breath escape from their lungs
   - If you have failed to replace the tracheostomy tube you should cover the tracheal stoma and provide rescue breaths by bag and mask (or mouth to mouth) if the patient has a patent upper airway or by mouth to stoma if the patient does not have a patent upper airway

   You will know your breathing has been effective if you can see the patient's chest rise and fall with each breath. After five breaths, you must check to see whether or not the patient has signs of life or a pulse
8. If there are no signs of life/pulse or you are not sure, you will need to perform chest compressions as well as providing the patient with ventilation breaths
9. Chest compressions should compress the lower half of the sternum. The rate for chest compressions is 100–120 per minute
10. Using two fingers for an infant and one or two hands for a patient, compress the lower half of the sternum 15 times by at least one-third of the diameter of the chest, and then give two ventilations
11. Give 1 minute of 15 chest compressions to two breaths and then call for help

If the patient recovers, place them in the recovery position, and continue to assess and support.

## 18.7 The ventilated patient

### Transport ventilators

Simple transport ventilators rely on oxygen pressure from the cylinder to drive the ventilator. Small transport ventilators such as Babypac™, Ventipac™ and Oxylog™ use differing volumes of oxygen depending on whether they are using 100% oxygen or entraining air. As a minimum, the ventilator will require the patient's minute volume of oxygen when delivering 100% oxygen. When air is entrained there may be some reduction in oxygen consumption, however it is always prudent to plan the need for 100% oxygen. Many ventilators will use at least an additional 1 l/min of oxygen as a 'driving gas' over and above that.

Setting up the ventilator may mean selecting the tidal volume and rate of ventilation (volume controlled) or selecting a suitable peak inspiratory pressure, inspiratory time and rate of ventilation (pressure controlled). The inspired oxygen concentration may be titrateable over a broad range (Babypac™) or may have two fixed values as provided by the Oxylog™, with air mix being approximately 50%.

Monitoring in basic models often involves no more than an airway pressure gauge; alarms are basic or even non-existent. Despite this, these ventilators are considered reliable and easy to use.

Advanced electronic circuitry in newer transport ventilators has enabled facilities such as the ability of the ventilator to synchronise with the breathing efforts of non-paralysed patients to be incorporated. The display and alarm systems are highly developed, but may need adjusting for paediatric use. Such technology requires electricity, and as a consequence these ventilators require a fully charged battery or mains supply. In addition, it is essential that the staff using this complex equipment should receive comprehensive education and training in the correct care and use of these state-of-the-art ventilators.

**The patient**

For the ventilated patient, oxygen consumption is dependent on minute volume and inspired oxygen requirement. The minute volume (MV) is calculated from the volume per breath (tidal volume or $V_t$) and the number of breaths a minute (respiratory rate or RR). In addition, 1 l/min oxygen is required as the driving gas. It should be noted that the driving gas has to be under pressure (about 10 bar) to enable the ventilator to function. Therefore, even though there may be some gas, under low pressure left in the cylinder, if the pressure falls below 10 bar the ventilator will cease to work.

**Minute volume (MV) = tidal volume ($V_t$) × respiratory rate (RR)**

Assuming that a patient may require 100% oxygen allows for deterioration en route and makes calculations simpler. If an adult patient has a tidal volume of 400 ml and a respiratory rate of 15 breaths per minute, then MV = 0.4 × 15 = 6 l/min. As the ventilator itself consumes 1 l/min, the total oxygen consumption is 7 l/min. For a neonate weighing 1500 g the tidal volume may be just 10 ml, with a respiratory rate of 60 breaths per minute; the MV would be 600 ml/min (0.6 l/min). As the ventilator itself consumes 1 l/min, the total oxygen consumption would be 1.6 l/min.

To calculate the oxygen requirement for the journey multiply the oxygen consumption in l/min by the total predicted length of the journey in minutes. Once this figure is obtained, double it.

Oxygen requirement (l) = 2 × oxygen consumption (l/min) × total journey time (min)

If the total volume required is less than a single cylinder, add a second cylinder to provide a back-up in case there is a mechanical failure of the first one.

**Always add a safety factor to cope with delays, breakdowns, etc. and 'double up' the predicted gas supply.**

**Always carry more than one cylinder of oxygen.**

**Formal training and education in the use of transport equipment should be regarded as mandatory.**

## 18.8 Summary

The patient with a difficult airway can be challenging to manage. The transportation of such a patient, whether the airway is secured or particularly if it is not secured, should only be undertaken by a team with the skills, equipment and training to deal with the potential problems that may present. It is vital that the consultant in charge is fully appraised of the situation at all times so that they can ensure appropriate support is provided to minimise the risks involved.

# CHAPTER 19
# Patient monitoring

---

**Learning outcomes**

After reading this chapter you will be able to:
- Describe the appropriate use of monitors in transfer
- Describe the monitoring of the ventilated patient

---

## 19.1 Introduction

When contemplating the transfer of any patient, either within a hospital or between different hospitals, the staff involved should consider how best to clinically observe the patient for signs of deterioration. The usefulness of basic clinical observations involving the triad of look, listen and feel cannot be overestimated. Basic monitoring of airway, breathing, circulation and consciousness must be applied every 15 minutes during all transfers regardless of duration, location and level of patient care required.

Basic observations may be difficult during the transfer of critically ill patients, but they do form a useful starting point during the initial assessment and a fall-back position when more complex systems of monitoring fail. Monitoring, using machine technology, is fraught with problems and clinical staff must be fully aware of the need to understand how monitoring works and its limitations. The application of monitoring must be a planned process; the most logical methodology is the use of the ABCDE approach.

## 19.2 Monitoring the patient

### Monitoring the airway

In the spontaneously breathing patient this can be undertaken simply by observing the ease with which the patient appears to be breathing. Look for signs of obstructed breathing – a 'seesaw' respiratory pattern or tracheal tug and recession in children – and listen for the tell-tale noisy stridor of an obstructed airway. In the ventilated patient, close observations of the airway pressure gauge and capnography should be used in conjunction with auscultation where appropriate.

### Monitoring of oxygenation and respiration

The basic observations of looking for cyanosis and counting the respiratory rate in the spontaneously breathing patient should not be forgotten. However, pulse oximetry should also be employed, and capnography must be used during the transport of all ventilated patients.

### Pulse oximetry

This uses light absorption as a means of estimating arterial oxygen saturation. It is based on the fact that oxyhaemoglobin and deoxyhaemoglobin absorb visible red and invisible infrared electromagnetic radiation differently. The oximeter sends a light signal through a vascular bed, such as a finger or an ear lobe, measures what is transmitted (or reflected) and then uses an algorithm to estimate the arterial oxygen saturation. As it is a mathematical prediction rather than a direct measurement, it is denoted as $SpO_2$ rather than $SaO_2$.

---

*Neonatal, Adult and Paediatric Safe Transfer and Retrieval: A Practical Approach to Transfers*, First Edition.
Edited by Bernard Foëx, Peter-Marc Fortune and Cassie Lawn.
© 2019 John Wiley & Sons Ltd. Published 2019 by John Wiley & Sons Ltd.

## Accuracy of pulse oximetry

Pulse oximetry estimates the oxygen saturation of haemoglobin which physiologically varies with partial pressure of oxygen in the blood ($PaO_2$). When changes in saturation are plotted against $PaO_2$ the resulting oxygen dissociation curve is sigmoid in shape and flat at high arterial oxygen levels. This means that a well oxygenated patient who has an $SpO_2$ of 100% may continue to show 100% saturation, whilst significant falls in $PaO_2$ occur.

As the $SpO_2$ reading falls below 90% the accuracy becomes less, and below 80% saturation the $SpO_2$ is at best a rough estimate with routine sensors. Because of these inaccuracies it is considered good practice to compare an $SpO_2$ reading recorded at the same time as an arterial blood gas $PaO_2$, if one is available.

Specialist sensors are available that deliver greater accuracy at lower levels of $SpO_2$ with some devices. These should be used, when available, for patients with cyanotic congenital heart conditions whose expected saturations will fall into a lower range.

---

**Remember:**
- **Oxygen saturation ($SpO_2$) is not the same as the $PaO_2$ as measured in arterial blood gases**
- **An $SpO_2$ value in the high 80s represents dangerously low values of $PaO_2$**
- **While a high $SpO_2$ indicates that the blood is well oxygenated, it does not mean that the ventilation is adequate**

---

## Limitations of pulse oximetry

Poor perfusion caused by reduced cardiac output, vasoconstriction or hypothermia can make it difficult to detect a reliable signal from a pulse oximeter probe, as can irregular heart rhthyms such as atrial fibrillation. Movement and vibration artefact can also result in unreliable readings. Such movement is inevitable during transport.

Strong ambient light, especially from fluorescent and xenon arc surgical lamps, can contaminate the signal from the probe, although most machines can now compensate for this effect. Nail varnish, especially if blue, green or black, can cause inaccurate $SpO_2$ readings. Acrylic nails do not in themselves affect pulse oximetry, although long fingernails can impede positioning of the probe on the finger.

Intravenous dyes such as methylene blue and indocyanine green can cause falsely low $SpO_2$ readings. Haemoglobinopathies may affect $SpO_2$ readings. High levels of carboxyhaemoglobin, which absorbs red light in a similar way as oxyhaemoglobin, may make the pulse oximeter overestimate the $SpO_2$ reading, therefore care should be taken in patients with smoke inhalation injury and carbon monoxide poisoning. High methaemoglobin levels also interfere with the accuracy of the $SpO_2$ readings, which tend to read 85%, regardless of the actual $SaO_2$.

## Setting up and using a pulse oximeter

As with any medical device, the user should have received formal training in the use and care of the equipment.

- Switch on the monitor and wait for it to complete the system self-test
- Select a probe that is compatible with the monitor, appropriate for the body part on which it is to be placed and suitable for the age and size of the patient
- Check that the probe is not damaged and secure it on the patient (finger, ear lobe or other body part, depending on the probe design). Pressure injury can result from incorrect positioning or prolonged attachment of the probe. Burns have been reported with probes that are incompatible with the oximeter or with inadequately protected probes in the high magnetic fields found in magnetic resonance scanners

Ensure that there is a good quality waveform before accepting the value of the $SpO_2$ as accurate. If the machine does not have a waveform display, check the intensity scale as an alternative, but much less reliable, quality control signal. Check that the heart rate is registered on the pulse oximeter; it should agree with that from the electrocardiogram (ECG). If not, this suggests an inadequate signal or machine error.

If the signal strength is low or the waveform is irregular, check that the probe is properly attached to the patient. If the problem cannot be attributed to poor peripheral perfusion or movement artefact, check that the probe gives a good signal with a regular waveform and a normal reading when you place the probe on yourself. A low $SpO_2$ may reflect a problem with the patient or with the monitor (measurement artefact). It is wise to assume that the problem lies with the patient but it is still important to check the waveform. Some causes of errors in pulse oximetry are listed in Box 19.1.

---

### Box 19.1 Causes of errors in pulse oximetry

- Cold/hypovolaemia/vasoconstriction
- Movement/vibration
- Non-invasive blood pressure (NIBP) cuff on same arm
- Ambient light
- Standard probes are unreliable under 85% saturation
- Presence of carboxyhaemoglobin or methaemoglobin

---

### End-tidal $CO_2$ monitoring (ETCO$_2$/capnography)

Capnography is the technique of measuring and displaying the carbon dioxide ($CO_2$) levels through the respiratory cycle (Figure 19.1). Carbon dioxide absorbs infrared radiation. The $CO_2$ level in the respiratory gas is measured by comparing how much infrared radiation is absorbed in a sampling chamber compared with a known source.

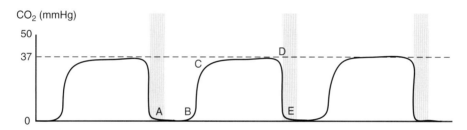

**Figure 19.1 The normal capnography – grey shaded areas represent inspiration**

During A-B, the first part of expiration, dead space gas from the airway endotracheal tube, trachea, bronchi and bronchioles (down to, but not including, the respiratory bronchioles and alveoli) is exhaled first (Figure 19.1). The capnography trace then rises (B-C) to a plateau (C-D) as the gas containing $CO_2$ from the alveoli and respiratory bronchioles is exhaled. During inspiration (D-E) the level of $CO_2$ in the sampling chamber falls rapidly.

In healthy individuals, the $CO_2$ level at the end of expiration (ETCO$_2$) approximates to the partial pressure of $CO_2$ as measured in arterial blood gases ($PaCO_2$).

The capnometer provides valuable supplementary evidence that the endotracheal tube is in the correct position. If the tube has been dislodged into the oesophagus, it registers no or minimal $CO_2$. It can also be used to monitor respiratory rate and serves to indicate when a circuit disconnection has occurred.

There are two types of capnometer. The sidestream capnometer sucks gas from the airway circuit through a fine bore tube via a water trap and the sample is analysed within the machine itself. The mainstream capnometer is situated within the airway circuit and tends to be bulkier and more vulnerable to damage.

#### Setting up and using a capnometer

1. All staff using the capnometer should be fully trained in its use
2. The capnometer should be calibrated at regular intervals according to the manufacturer's instructions
3. If using a mainstream capnometer, check that the sensor holder is patent and that the sensor panels are clean and not cracked

4. If using a sidestream capnometer, visually check the sampling tubing for signs of moisture and ensure that the water trap is empty
5. Switch on and allow a warm-up time with sensors attached to the breathing circuit
6. Ensure that the sensor or sampling tube is not lying lower than the endotracheal tube, so as to reduce the risk of secretions or condensation contaminating the sensor or blocking the tubing
7. Position the sensor or sampling tube to avoid traction on the endotracheal tube
8. Ensure that all airway connections are secure

### *Limitations of capnometry*

The $ETCO_2$ value may not be an accurate reflection of the $PaCO_2$ in the shocked patient.

Increased physiological dead space in the lungs caused by poor perfusion of upper (less dependent) parts of the lungs, results in expired gas with a lower $CO_2$ than from those areas that equilibrate well with blood flowing through the lungs. In such circumstances, the $ETCO_2$ is often less than the $PaCO_2$ and an arterial blood gas sample is needed to determine the true figure.

Correlating the $PaCO_2$ and $ETCO_2$ before setting off on a transfer is helpful in maintaining control en route, but great care must be taken in interpreting changes in the $ETCO_2$ if there are concomitant changes in the circulatory status (Box 19.2).

---

**Box 19.2 Check the end-tidal $CO_2$ against the arterial $PaCO_2$**

A reduced $ETCO_2$ may be due to hyperventilation, or it may be due to ventilation/perfusion mismatch caused by:

- Hypovolaemia
- Sepsis
- Heart failure
- Pulmonary embolism

---

Capnography should be monitored in all intubated and ventilated patients. A high $ETCO_2$ generally indicates underventilation and requires an increase in minute ventilation. In neonatal patients higher values are often acceptable.

Increasing $ETCO_2$ may relate to a problem with inadequate ventilator settings or to partial airway obstruction (e.g. secretions). Other causes include an increase in temperature or metabolic rate (Figure 19.2).

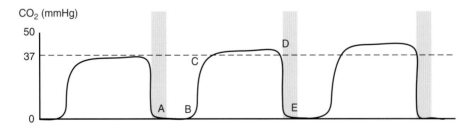

**Figure 19.2 Capnograph showing increasing $ETCO_2$**

A falling $ETCO_2$ indicates overventilation or a fall in temperature or metabolic rate (Figure 19.3).

The $ETCO_2$ may continue to slope upwards during late expiration, with loss of the plateau. This occurs when the airway or ventilator tubing becomes obstructed or bronchospasm develops (Figure 19.4).

If the patient is attempting to breathe on a portable ventilator, this may be revealed by dips on the plateau of the waveform, the so-called 'curare cleft' (Figure 19.5).

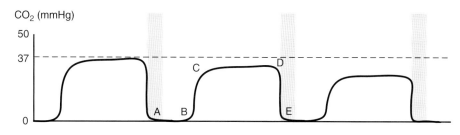

**Figure 19.3 Capnograph showing decreasing ETCO$_2$**

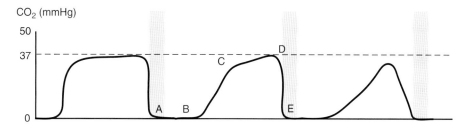

**Figure 19.4 Capnograph showing loss of a plateau**

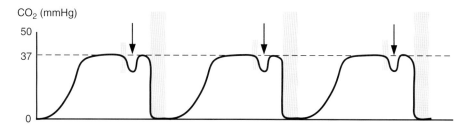

**Figure 19.5 Capnograph showing 'curare cleft' attempted breathing**

Excessive damping or flattening of the waveform may indicate blockage of the suction tubing in a sidestream capnometer. On the other hand, contamination of a mainstream sensor by secretions may cause the ETCO$_2$ to be overestimated. High respiratory rates (>30/min) may preclude accurate measurement of ETCO$_2$, especially in sidestream capnometers. The fall in barometric pressure at an altitude can result in an underestimate of ETCO$_2$, unless the machine has a built-in altimeter to make corrections.

As in pulse oximetry, the waveform serves as a quality control signal from which to judge the reliability of the readings. If the function of the capnometer is in doubt, test it yourself, by exhaling into the sampling port to confirm a normal waveform with an expected ETCO$_2$ of 5.0–5.6 kPa (38–42 mmHg).

## 19.3 Monitoring the ventilated patient during transportation

Monitoring of the ventilated patient is a complex process involving the need to observe a number of individual components:

- The patient's chest for signs of equal sided movement, synchronous with the ventilator
- The patient's breathing system connections
- State of the oxygen supply
- Pulse oximeter display
- Capnography display
- Ventilator display, gauges and settings

## Monitoring the cardiovascular system

Some basic observations are not really practical during transfer of patients; however, for short journeys at strategic intervals, for example, some basic observations can be quickly carried out to ensure that all is well, e.g. whilst waiting for a lift. The pulse can be assessed in terms of its rate, rhythm and quality and the capillary refill time observed to mark peripheral perfusion. Over a longer period of time, the urine output is often a useful index of major organ perfusion.

### *The electrocardiogram*

The ECG is well established as a monitoring tool and provides useful information about heart rate and arrhythmias. The ECG trace may also have a limited role in detecting ischaemia. By placing the electrodes in the CM5 position, left ventricular ischaemia may be detected more readily (Figure 19.6).

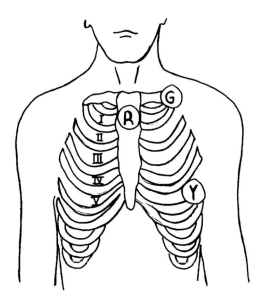

**Figure 19.6  CM5 positioning of ECG leads**

Effective monitoring and interpretation of the ECG trace during the transfer of any patient, particularly small children, may be made difficult by artefacts. Despite the use of modern artefact rejection monitors, problems are often encountered. High frequency filters reduce distortions from muscle movement, mains current and electromagnetic interference from other equipment. The low frequency filters reduce respiratory and transfer induced body movement artefacts.

The silver/chloride electrodes need to have the best possible electrical connection between the electrode and the skin.

- The correct storage of electrodes is vitally important; the conducting gel must be allowed to dry out
- In adult patients gentle dermabrasion of the layer of non-conductive dead epithelial cells with gauze may improve contact
- Placing electrodes over bony prominences will reduce artefacts from muscle movement

Shielding of cables and leads helps to reduce interference from high frequency (AC mains) and radiofrequency induced currents. This shielding consists of electroconductive woven material which is 'earthed'; any interference currents are induced in the metal screen and not in the monitoring leads. However, the 'flying leads' leading to the electrodes have much less shielding. It is therefore good practice to prevent these leads from moving especially during transfer; a hypoallergenic tape can be used to strap them onto the patient's chest.

> **Careful attention paid to electrode storage and application will help to reduce ECG artefacts.**

### Blood pressure measurement

The measurement of blood pressure by manual sphygmomanometry has largely been replaced by automated blood pressure measuring devices. Such NIBP machines offer advantages of convenience and reduced inter-observer error. NIBP has a role in the intra-hospital transportation of non-critically ill patients. However, in inter-hospital transportation medicine, the major disadvantages include motion artefact and the rapid loss of battery power due to the power consumption of the pneumatic pump. Invasive arterial monitoring is generally recommended for the transportation of the critically ill with NIBP considered as a back-up system. However, if a transfer is time critical, the delay in establishing an arterial line may necessitate the use of NIBP alone.

### Invasive arterial pressure monitoring

Arterial pressure may be conveniently measured on a beat-to-beat basis using an intra-arterial cannula attached to a transducer. The transducer converts the physical pressure wave into an electrical signal, which is amplified and displayed by the monitor. The radial artery is the preferred site for the cannula, although femoral, dorsalis pedis and brachial artery sites are possible alternatives. Additionally, an umbilical arterial line may be sited in neonates. In order to keep the system patent, intra-arterial lines should be continually flushed at 0.5–3 ml/h with saline or heparinised saline delivered by either a pressure bag system or syringe driver.

As with the pulse oximeter and capnometer, the displayed waveform contains invaluable information and serves as a quality check, helping to identify both clinical and technical problems.

### Setting up and using invasive arterial pressure monitoring

1. The saline flush system should be prepared. Not all hospitals continue the practice of heparinising the saline with 1000 IU heparin per litre
2. The tubing should be short and non-compliant, and the number of three-way taps minimised, so as not to distort the waveform
3. Ensure that all connections are tight, that there are no bubbles within the system and that the flush bag is pressurised
4. Connect the indwelling cannula to the tubing and flush manually. Check the arterial waveform
5. Secure the transducer at the level of the fourth intercostal space in the mid-axillary line
6. 'Zero' the transducer according to the monitor's instructions, with the three-way tap open to atmosphere and to the transducer. Return the three-way tap to the in-line position to display the waveform and readings

### Clinical problems

It is important to remember that a normal blood pressure does not necessarily indicate adequate cardiac output.

The waveform may indicate clinical problems; a spiky waveform with a short systolic time is seen in hypovolaemia. An arterial trace that seems to swing with respiration is associated with hypovolaemia, so-called 'pre-load responsiveness'. Confirmation of this should be obtained from other observations, especially if the patient has significant airway obstruction (asthma) or is being ventilated with high pressures. The waveform may also reveal technical problems, such as a resonant, overshooting trace or a flattened, overdamped trace. In such cases it is worth rechecking for bubbles and leaks, checking that the flush bag is still pressurised and flushing the line manually. Consider removing any unnecessary three-way taps or excessive tubing. Consider re-zeroing and comparing the readings with NIBP values in the event of unexpected values, but do not simply ascribe abnormalities to monitor dysfunction. It is more likely that the fault lies with the patient, who may need urgent attention. Re-zero periodically during prolonged transfers.

## Invasive central venous pressure monitoring

With the advent of central venous catheters comprising four and more lumens, some might argue that there is less need for large bore peripheral lines; however, central venous lines can become dislodged, thus losing one or all lumens. You should work on the basis that the worst case scenario occurs – the line migrates.

## Cardiac output monitoring

Currently many of the techniques for computing and displaying cardiac output are not compatible with the transport of critically ill patients.

**Monitoring the nervous system**

Basic clinical skills involving close observation of the patient's reaction to stimuli and compliance with treatment form the mainstay of neurological monitoring. In the conscious patient this is not difficult. However, many critically ill patients being transferred are sedated and paralysed. The clinician is therefore reliant on surrogate measures of awareness and pain such as pulse rate, blood pressure and the presence of sweating. Pupil size and reaction may be especially relevant in the brain injured patient.

## 19.4  Power supplies – batteries and inverters

Reports of critical care equipment failure during transfer occur with frightening regularity, many of which are due to battery failure. Staff involved in transfer medicine rely on power supplies almost as much as they do on oxygen. There are two types of battery in current use – rechargeable and non-rechargeable (Table 19.1).

| Table 19.1  Common types of batteries | |
| --- | --- |
| **Type** | **Construction** |
| Non-rechargeable | Zinc carbon, zinc chloride and alkaline batteries |
| Rechargeable | Nickel cadmium (NiCd), nickel metal hydride (NiMh), lithium ion (Li ion) and sealed lead acid (SLA) |

One of the most important observed differences between non-rechargeable and rechargeable batteries is their discharge characteristics. Figure 19.7 contrasts a non-rechargeable alkaline battery with a rechargeable NiCd battery. The alkaline battery power output deteriorates slowly, whereas the NiCd battery loses power over a few minutes.

In general, rechargeable batteries do not store as much energy as non-rechargeable batteries; however, SLA batteries are used in some heavy duty applications.

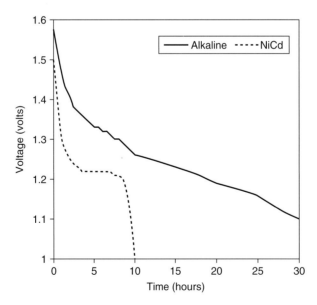

**Figure 19.7  Discharge curves for AA size batteries – in both cases the discharge current is 60 mA. Contrasts between a non-rechargeable alkaline battery and a rechargeable NiCd battery.** Reproduced with permission from Medical Devices Agency

## 19.5  Summary

Some science behind the use of oxygen and monitors may help to understand how to use this equipment to the best advantage.

CHAPTER 20

# The infectious or contaminated patient

---

**Learning outcomes**

After reading this chapter, you will be able to:
- Define the essential differences between infectious and chemically contaminated patients
- Describe the structured approach to the safe management of the infectious patient
- Describe how to assess the risk of a patient being infectious
- Outline the principles of ACCEPT can assist safe transfers

---

## 20.1 Introduction

There is currently a heightened awareness of the risks of infection transmission both to staff and to other patients. Infectious patients continue to pose a threat to others until the infection is eradicated. During a hospital admission, an infectious patient may require transfer within the hospital or even to a specialist centre in another hospital. Such transfers expose healthcare workers to the ongoing risk of infection transmission.

Contaminated patients are usually those who have been exposed to some form of chemical released as a result of an accidental spillage outside the hospital. Such patients pose a threat only to those who have close physical contact. Once properly decontaminated, the threat disappears, and it becomes safe to transfer these patients according to their medical needs.

## 20.2 The potentially infectious patient

Standard precautions, or what used to be called universal precautions, should remind healthcare staff that all patients should be regarded as potential sources of infections, which may be transmitted to the staff or between patients.

The transfer of the infectious or contaminated patient is usually a primary transfer from a residence, or the scene of an incident, to the hospital's emergency department. Once admitted, it is rare for patients to undergo a secondary transfer to another hospital, except where specific medical treatment at a tertiary specialist centre is indicated. However, infectious patients will have to be transferred safely within the hospital from the dmergency department to an appropriate location within the hospital.

---

**When dealing with cases of unusual illness, which may be infectious or as a result of contamination, the welfare of staff and other patients is paramount; the emphasis is on prevention of transmission (Table 20.1).**

---

*Neonatal, Adult and Paediatric Safe Transfer and Retrieval: A Practical Approach to Transfers*, First Edition.
Edited by Bernard Foëx, Peter-Marc Fortune and Cassie Lawn.
© 2019 John Wiley & Sons Ltd. Published 2019 by John Wiley & Sons Ltd.

**Table 20.1** Details of several modes of transmission of infection

| Transmission route | Involves |
| --- | --- |
| Direct contact | Direct transmission of body fluids |
| Indirect contact | Indirect transmission of body fluids via an intermediate agent: personnel, equipment, hard surfaces |
| Droplets | Aerosol droplet spread (not usually more than 1 m) |
| Airborne | Small particles (5 microns or less) or infected dust, may travel long distances depending on airflows |

An ABC approach to the safety aspects of infection control has been suggested. In order to avoid confusion and for the purposes of this book, these will be referred to as **a b c d** as in Table 20.2.

**Table 20.2** The **a b c d** approach to the safety aspects of infection control

| Title | Description |
| --- | --- |
| **a** Alert | Be alert to the possibility of transmissible disease |
| **b** Barrier | Use barrier precautions (physical separation and personal protective equipment) |
| **c** Clean and disinfect | Ensure all potentially contaminated equipment and surfaces are cleaned and disinfected |
| **d** Dispose | Ensure safe handling and disposal of all waste |

Linking this in with the ACCEPT structure gives the following structure.

## A – Assessment

- What is the problem?
- What is being/should be done?
- What is the effect of these actions?
- What is needed next?

The *problem* is that any patient may pose an infection risk. Following the outbreaks of, for example, severe acute respiratory syndrome (SARS), swine flu, Ebola and Middle East respiratory syndrome coronavirus (MERS CoV), a general state of heightened awareness of the possibility of an epidemic of life-threatening viral illnesses exists. Staff in emergency departments are advised to be **a** (alert) to the possibility that a patient presenting with an unusual illness may be the index case for an outbreak.

The following enquiries should be made:

- Where:
  - have the patients been recently?
  - do they live?
  - do they work?
- Have they travelled anywhere?
- How did they travel?

Mechanisms are in place to **a** (alert) those in the front line to any emerging pattern of increases in reported infections. In the UK, the Health Protection Agency (HPA) is charged with coordinating health protection across the UK. The Communicable Disease Surveillance Centre (CDSC), which is part of the HPA, receives information and coordinates the dissemination of surveillance intelligence. Other sources of information include Eurosurveillance; weekly updates distributed as Communicable Disease Report Weekly (CDR Weekly); and, if necessary, alerts are e-mailed out to key personnel in hospital and primary care trusts. In effect the HPA acts as a barometer of the spread of infectious diseases not only in the UK but anywhere in the world (Figure 20.1).

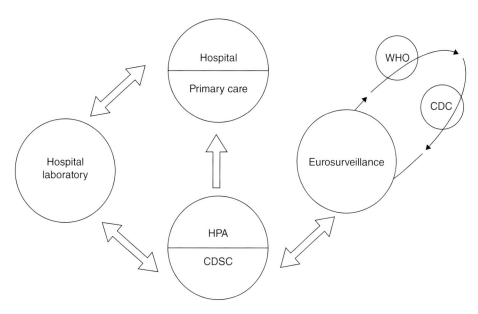

**Figure 20.1 UK communicable disease surveillance and alerting systems.** CDC, Centers for Disease Control and Prevention; CDSC, Communicable Disease Surveillance Centre; HPA, Health Protection Agency; WHO, World Health Organisation

With this high index of suspicion, appropriate safety measures can be implemented early. *What should be done* in terms of safety is to institute **b** (barrier) precautions. These will include immediate physical isolation of the patient, restriction of the number of staff coming into contact with the patient and institution of appropriate personal protective equipment (PPE) measures. The *effect* of correct application of these measures should be to reduce the risk to staff and other patients. What is needed *next* is a safe transfer to an appropriate location.

During the assessment and initial treatment stages, appropriate life-saving treatment should be instituted as required, with due regard to personal safety. However, procedures requiring close contact should only be carried out with appropriate protection. Procedures likely to cause an increase in loss of body fluids or aerosolisation should be strictly limited to those which cannot wait until the patient is located in a more secure environment. It is also advisable to limit the transport of patients to essential medical investigations only, and for patients to wear high efficiency masks during transport. (Note, however, that to ensure high quality diagnosis, especially for the first cases detected, X-rays should be performed in the X-ray department rather than by mobile machine wherever possible.)

## C – Control

During the assessment, the team leader should allocate the task of 'safety controller' to someone until the arrival of an infection control specialist. Tasks will consist of:

- **b** (barrier) controlling access to the quarantined area
- **b** (barrier) compliance with the correct PPE procedures
- **d** (dispose) correct disposal of contaminated items
- **c** (clean and disinfect) thorough cleaning and disinfection of the area and any equipment used during the transfer

## C – Communicate

Using a structured approach, communication with the following people is required:

- The senior consultant responsible for the care of the patient
- Hospital management
- The infection control team in the trust
- The laboratories that 'high risk' specimens will be sent to
- The local medical microbiologist and chemical pathologist
- The local consultant in communicable disease control

### E – Evaluation

The *need* to transfer the patient to a secure environment will be agreed. In most cases this will be an intra-hospital transfer. The competencies of accompanying staff will be dictated by the clinical needs of the patient as well as the ability to ensure that infection transmission is minimised. Should it be imperative that an inter-hospital transfer is undertaken, appropriate arrangements should be made with the ambulance service. Helicopters and private transport must not be used.

### P – Preparation and packaging

Patient and staff packaging must ensure that all reasonable measures are taken to ensure that any potential contamination of the staff, the transfer equipment, and the environment is reduced to a minimum. These are **b** (barrier) precautions.

### T – Transportation and handover

During the transfer, the team must remain **a** (alert) to the possibility of a breach in the protective measures taken to limit contamination. Following handover, all equipment must be thoroughly **c** (cleaned and disinfected); disposable PPE equipment must be removed, taking care not to contaminate clean areas; this equipment must be **d** (disposed) of in a safe manner. Finally, a record of all staff who have been in contact with the patient should be made and passed to the infection control officer.

## 20.3  The potentially contaminated patient

Twenty first century lifestyle depends on technology and chemicals. Each year over 49 million tonnes of chemicals are transported around the UK. The manufacture, storage and transportation of the most toxic chemicals are subject to stringent controls; however, accidents do happen. There is, of course, also the constant worry about the deliberate release of chemicals into a public place.

Emergency services work together to develop contingency plans to respond rapidly to contain chemical incidents. The HPA is also involved in supporting the NHS in such emergency situations. These chemical, biological, radiological and nuclear defense (CBRN) plans cover a wide range of possible scenarios. There are two main categories of chemical incident based on the speed of development of the incident:

*Category I incident.* In a category I incident (where the presentation is acute, and a chemical or toxic aetiology is most likely) decontamination is crucial in preventing secondary contamination. This will also be important in suspected overt deliberate release of biological agents and where cases may have been exposed to, for example, unidentified powders or gases.

*Category II incident.* For a category II incident (where presentations may be more delayed and biological agents are rather more likely) the situation is more complicated because of the manner in which patients might present. Although healthcare staff may be pre-warned of the arrival of cases of unusual illness, it is also possible that the healthcare staff will be the ones recognising the unusual nature of the presentation. As soon as there is any suspicion of an unusual aetiology, all staff should take precautions to protect themselves, primarily from biological agents (as above), although decontamination might once again be appropriate if the clinical picture is suggestive of chemical exposure.

> **Only clean, or decontaminated, casualties should be transported to hospital by ambulance.**

One of the primary functions of the emergency services response to an acute chemical (category I) incident is decontaminating those who are likely to have been contaminated. This involves the difficult task of preventing the public from leaving the scene of the incident without decontamination.

Despite their best efforts, some people escape the cordon, only to present themselves at hospital later. It is worth noting that many of the casualties following the 1994 Tokyo nerve agent (sarin gas) attack occurred at the receiving hospitals. This is because no early decontamination took place at the scene, no PPE was worn in the initial stages and no control was placed on contaminated members of the general public. Self-referrals added to the problem, a situation which is likely to be the case within the UK. On entry to the warm hospital environment, the contaminated casualties began to 'off gas', thus contaminating those medical professionals attempting to save their lives.

Decontamination of self-referrals is a hospital NHS trust responsibility. There is likely to be some prior warning that casualties will arrive in an emergency department and cases should have been decontaminated prior to transfer to hospital. If this has not been performed then it should be done immediately on arrival at hospital. Specialist decontamination techniques are taught on training courses such as HAZIMMS.

## Types of contamination

The modes of chemical contamination (Table 20.3) are similar to those described in Table 20.1.

| Table 20.3  Modes of chemical contamination | |
| --- | --- |
| **Transmission route** | **Involves** |
| Direct contact | Primary contamination |
| Droplets | Primary contamination |
| Airborne | Primary contamination |
| Indirect contact | Secondary contamination; contamination by another person |

There are two main types of exposure to a contaminant:

- *Primary contamination.* Exposure where the contaminated person was in the vicinity of the agent when it was released. Any person who has suffered primary contamination must be thoroughly decontaminated
- *Secondary contamination.* Exposure where a person has come into contact with an individual who has suffered primary exposure prior to decontamination

## Transfer

The issue of the possible inter-hospital transfer of a chemically contaminated patient should not arise, as patients with significant injuries warranting transfer to a tertiary centre will almost certainly have been brought to the hospital by the ambulance service, who will have decontaminated them at scene. However, some patients with minor injuries, which still warrant admission, may self-present. These patients, if identified as potentially contaminated, must be decontaminated outside the emergency department prior to admission and transfer to a ward.

## 20.4  Summary

It is important to distinguish between infectious and chemically contaminated patients. Applying a structured approach to safety through the ACCEPT sequence is vitally important to prevent the transmission of infectious diseases to healthcare workers and other patients. Alert staff, who make the best use of barrier precautions, will help to prevent the spread of infectious diseases during the transfer process. The chemically contaminated patient must be decontaminated prior to any transfer.

# CHAPTER 21
# Governance, legal and insurance issues

---

## Learning outcomes

After reading this chapter, you will be able to discuss key issues during transfers pertaining to:
- Clinical governance
- Legal and litigation matters
- Vicarious liability
- Accident insurance

---

## 21.1 Introduction

The principles of clinical governance have been embraced by healthcare professionals since the inception of the NHS in 1948. However, its delivery within the UK was only structured and formalised more recently. Clinical governance is now firmly embedded in all areas of practice and applies to all staff working in healthcare.

Hospital staff need to have a clear understanding of the legal framework within which they operate for their own, the patients' and the organisation's benefit. Medico-legal issues are by their nature both varied and complex and litigation is on the rise. This chapter reviews the key legal issues that should be understood when undertaking inter-hospital transport. These discussions are by no means definitive and should not be relied upon for specific legal concerns: in such cases expert advice should always be sought through the local trust's legal department.

The nature of the process of inter-hospital transfer exposes the patient, the staff and the public to an enhanced level of risk. The possibility of sustaining an injury, secondary to an accident, whilst undertaking inter-hospital transfers is only too real. The insurance cover provided for transport staff is not standardised and it can be extremely difficult to ascertain the details of cover within any particular trust. Best practice is to provide additional insurance provision for staff involved in transport activities.

## 21.2 Clinical governance

Clinical governance was formalised out of the need for accountability for the safe delivery of health services. At its inception in 1998 it was defined in the consultation document *A First Class Service: Quality in the New NHS* as:

> *A framework through which NHS organisations are accountable for continuously improving the quality of their services and safeguarding high standards of care by creating an environment in which excellence in clinical care will flourish.*

A common model used to illustrate the principle components of clinical governance is the seven pillars of excellence supported by five foundation stones as shown in Box 21.1.

---

*Neonatal, Adult and Paediatric Safe Transfer and Retrieval: A Practical Approach to Transfers*, First Edition.
Edited by Bernard Foëx, Peter-Marc Fortune and Cassie Lawn.
© 2019 John Wiley & Sons Ltd. Published 2019 by John Wiley & Sons Ltd.

---

**Box 21.1 Components of clinical governance**

*Seven pillars of governance*
- Clinical effectiveness
- Risk management effectiveness
- Patient experience
- Communication effectiveness
- Resource effectiveness
- Strategic effectiveness
- Learning effectiveness

*Five foundation stones*
- Systems awareness
- Teamwork
- Communication
- Ownership
- Leadership

---

The key government bodies associated with this process have changed their titles several times in recent years. Currently they comprise of the National Institute for Health and Care Excellence (NICE), the Care Quality Commission (CQC) and the Clinical Governance Support Team (CGST). These bodies are involved in regulation and facilitation of the delivery of good clinical governance in partnership with the NHS workforce.

It is fundamentally important to appreciate that clinical governance is the responsibility of each and every employee of the NHS, both clinical and non-clinical. This means that it is up to each of us to ensure the delivery of a safe, high quality service at all times. For those of us engaged in transport medicine, the planning and delivery of local service provision will require a risk assessment, proactive planning and constant audit to ensure the delivery of a high quality, safe service and ongoing quality improvement.

For each area, or 'pillar', there are specific standards against which trusts are judged and held accountable. For instance, safety issues (see Chapter 12) are assessed against current health and safety legislation and other appropriate guidance and legislation. Clinical governance processes should ensure that probity, patient safety, quality assurance and quality improvement are all core components of healthcare activities. This is best achieved through the promotion of a proactive culture where service delivery is well structured with clear managerial and clinical leadership. Individual accountability is also a fundamental component of a good governance process but must be delivered within a no-blame culture that recognises that it is more often processes than individuals that lead to poor or unsafe practice (see Chapter 4).

A safety and quality management system should be in place to assist teams in following a formal process when planning, implementing and evaluating activities within the governance framework. An example of this would be a regular, formal review of clinical incidents at which a representative from each staff group should be present to ensure a balanced view. Any learning gained from this review should be widely shared in order to promote quality improvement and prevent future occurrence.

## 21.3 Transport lead personnel

A medical and nursing lead clinician should always be identified with overall responsibility for directing the transport service. These roles should include management of guidelines, staffing, staff training, equipment provision and service level agreements. The director or an appropriate identified deputy must be contactable at all times for professional guidance on any problems. This individual is the clinical governance lead for the service.

## 21.4 Staff training

Trusts with a designated transport service must ensure that the staff who undertake transport duties have appropriate training. They must be able to demonstrate their competence and experience in clinical care, appropriate to the patients being transferred, specifically in the transport setting. Appropriate training should prepare staff to efficiently and safely manage the logistical aspects of transport and to prepare, use and troubleshoot the equipment employed. Staff must also be familiar with all the relevant documentation and guidelines. A formal competency assessment should be regularly completed for all clinical staff. Formal documentation should be completed for each assessment and signed by both the assessor and the assessee. This then serves as a record that training has been undertaken and completed satisfactorily.

## 21.5 Vicarious liability

Every practitioner has a duty of care to their patients. Organisationally, the NHS has an overall duty to ensure that healthcare is delivered to a minimum standard. The operational realisation of that duty is delegated to local healthcare trusts. Each trust's chief executive carries responsibility for the maintenance of standards within the trust. Theoretically, they are ultimately responsible for the actions and omissions of all staff employed by the trust. This responsibility is known as vicarious liability.

The chief executive and their team will seek to ensure appropriate professional development for all clinical staff in order to ensure quality. Providing staff act reasonably, and within their competence, the chief executive will honour their responsibility for vicarious liability for all work undertaken on behalf of the trust wherever that work takes place. This includes work undertaken whilst transferring a patient to or from another hospital. It is important to note that if staff are judged to have acted unreasonably, and outside their competence or normal scope of practice, the trust may not consider itself responsible for the effects of the acts and omissions of these staff. The staff themselves may find themselves liable.

Where transport teams operate across one or more trusts this becomes more complicated. Whilst all of the above remains true, there is also a responsibility to raise concerns should the team encounter suboptimal or unsafe practice. Generally such concerns are relatively low level and can be addressed through outreach teaching. However, serious concerns should be raised formally through appropriate communications at a senior level between trusts.

## 21.6 Negligence

When there is a perception, from any quarter, that things have gone wrong, there may be allegations of negligence. Legal proof of negligence requires the fulfilment of specific criteria. To prove a case of negligence the following must be established:

- A duty of care existed
- There was a failure of that duty of care
- That the patient suffered some harm
- A chain of causation can be demonstrated which links all three of the above

Unless all the above criteria are established, negligence cannot be proven. A failure to thoroughly document the care of a patient, particularly if there is an untoward event, may seriously harm your defence!

## 21.7 Record keeping

A contemporaneous record of all the key events of a transfer episode should be made. This should start with the details of the initial conversation requesting transfer and cover the entire time through to the handover to the receiving hospital staff, or the decision not to transfer. All communications, face to face or via telephone should be documented and where possible recorded. Independent or regional transport services, which are not based at the receiving intensive care unit, should keep their own copies of the transport record and provide copies at the point of handover to the receiving unit. One copy must always be filed in the patient's hospital in-patient record. These records must be stored by both the hospital, and the transport service in this instance, for the recommended statutory period (currently 25 years for children and 8 years from conclusion of treatment in adults).

In addition to written documentation, some transport services also use a telephone recording system. This records all calls initiated or received through the identified telephone lines/extensions. All callers must be made aware of the recording system, either with a pre-recorded message prior to the call being answered or by the staff member answering the call. Likewise, if a conference calling facility is used, each additional individual joining the call should be introduced to ensure all parties are aware of who is participating in the conversation. These telephone recordings must be downloaded and stored in the same way as documented records, for the same statutory period.

## 21.8 Accountability

The referring consultant in charge of the patient's care will remain responsible for their care until the transfer team have received the handover, assessed the patient and formally accepted the patient into their care. Thereafter the responsibility for clinical care ultimately rests with the consultant in charge of the team undertaking the transfer. However, the boundaries are often blurred. The transfer team will usually recommend a management plan to be followed prior to their arrival. This would be considered expert advice. Assuming that the advice is followed, the lead consultant of the transfer team will then take some responsibility for the consequences of their advice being followed. Where advice is not followed and a poor outcome occurs it will be for the local team to explain why they took an alternative course (appropriately or otherwise). In such a case the transport team may be required to demonstrate they gave appropriate advice. In the absence of such evidence an expert team might be criticised for not providing appropriate guidance.

There may be a particularly difficult period during stabilisation, preparation and packaging where a junior grade transport doctor is working under the scrutiny of a local consultant. Again, clear communication and accurate documentation is key. Usually the local team will be very supportive and it is advisable for transport teams to use all available resources. They should request senior local support as appropriate. For example, a paediatric middle grade transport doctor should request the help of a consultant anaesthetist from the referring hospital if an intubation is expected to be difficult.

The boundaries of clinical responsibility become particularly blurred when dealing with specialist referrals. For instance, a referring hospital may receive advice from the specialist centre that may indicate a course of treatment should be started prior to transfer. The question arises as to who is responsible for the care of the patient prior to transfer; is it the referring medical team or is it the receiving specialist medical team that is offering advice? A simple example may be a head injured patient in one hospital being referred to a neurosciences centre at another hospital; the neurosciences hospital recommends 500 ml of 20% mannitol, the referring hospital declines to administer this and there is a subsequent legal argument as to who was responsible for the poor outcome of the patient. There is currently no legislation as to who takes majority accountability during these periods of joint care.

When the situation requires the referring hospital to undertake the inter-hospital transfer, it is not uncommon for the medical or surgical teams to ask the anaesthetic service to manage the transfer. The lines of responsibility will alter between teams in the same way as would occur using an external transfer service for specialist referrals. The local team, the anaesthetic team and the receiving (specialist) centre will all assume some part of the responsibility of care. Therefore the structured approach described in this manual should be followed especially with regard to handover and documentation that may be minimal or even omitted in these circumstances.

The use of a standard operating procedure by transport teams provides clarity of both responsibility and the process for all those involved.

Negligence claims in respect of morbidity and mortality will have to prove the likely origin (time and place) of the act or omission that resulted in injury in order to apportion blame correctly. In other words, a receiving hospital cannot be held responsible for an act or omission that occurred before it was contacted and does not assume the greater part of the responsibility until the patient is fully handed over and accepted into their team's care.

## 21.9 Death during transport

The transport consultant should always be involved in any decision to move a patient that the transport clinicians consider to be at a high risk of dying. Normally there should be a discussion at consultant level by the referring and transport team to ensure it is appropriate to move the patient. The situation and risks should be explained to the patient (where possible) and/ or the parents/family (as appropriate) and they should be given an opportunity to question the decisions taken. If the patient's or family's opinion is at odds with that held by the professionals then the usual processes governing consent should come into play in order to guide further actions. Telephone conference call facilities may enable all parties to be simultaneously involved in the discussion, enhancing clarity and transparency. These discussions and the decision taken must be thoroughly documented in the clinical notes. If any person disagrees with the chosen course this should be documented, together with their reasons for disagreeing where possible.

Should the patient die during transfer the exact location of the death will determine which coroner should receive the initial referral of the case. If it is an international ground transfer the exact location determines jurisdiction. However, if it is an air transfer the pilot must be notified as the designation of the airspace and nationality of the airline may affect the decision of where to land under international aviation law.

## 21.10 Advance care plans and 'do not attempt cardiopulmonary resuscitation' orders

In some circumstances the transport team may be requested to transport a patient with a 'do not attempt cardiopulmonary resuscitation' (DNACPR) order or an advance care plan (ACP). The decision to transfer in the context of DNACPR must be made jointly between the referring, receiving and transport staff at consultant level, and must include the consent of the patient, parent or family (as appropriate). This decision, including details of any appropriate interventions, must be documented and signed in the clinical notes of both the referring hospital and the transport notes. Some ACPs may contain sufficient detail in this regard and may be used as the master document for guidance.

## 21.11 Disability and disablement entitlement/insurance cover

All NHS staff are entitled to benefit from the NHS injury benefits scheme. There is no qualifying period: everyone is covered from the day they join the NHS. The scheme is not part of the NHS pension scheme; it is governed by different rules. It covers all NHS employees and general practitioners, whether or not they are members of the NHS pension scheme.

The NHS injury benefits scheme provides a spectrum of benefits to the employee, in relation to temporary or permanent inability to work, up to and including death. In essence, the benefits are based on the present salary of the employee, years of service and, in the case of death, any dependants. These benefits are subject to a form of means test and may be curtailed if other compensation for the injury or benefits from other sources are being paid out. NHS trusts do subscribe to what is commonly known as employer's liability insurance schemes.

The NHS Litigation Authority is the insurance broker for NHS trusts. Details of benefits which may be obtained from this scheme are not clear. What is clear is that some form of negligence on the part of the employer may have to be proved, and the maximum compensation is rather limited.

As a result of the formation of the NHS Litigation Authority, NHS trusts are technically no longer permitted to enrol their staff in personal accident insurance schemes. Following this ruling the Intensive Care Society (UK) and Paediatric Intensive Care Society arranged personal accident insurance for their members. This comprehensive insurance package is available to all members of these societies. Membership of the Association of Anaesthetists of Great Britain and Ireland (AAGBI) confers similar benefits. The common belief amongst nursing staff that membership of the Royal College of Nursing (RCN) confers automatic personal accident insurance benefits is wholly untrue: the RCN will, however, arrange introduction to an approved insurance broker.

## 21.12 Summary

Clinical governance provides a structure to deliver continual improvement and high quality, safe medical care.

Transport medicine is a complex area. An understanding of the principles of vicarious liability and clinical negligence illustrate the importance of following the formal structures and approaches described in this manual. By following these principles our patients should receive the best care possible and, should an untoward event occur, the clinical staff would receive all appropriate support through their trust and the legal system.

Staff undertaking inter-hospital transfers are advised that they should check that adequate financial arrangements are in place for themselves and their dependants in the event of an accident.

# CHAPTER 22
# Documentation

---

## Learning outcomes

After reading this chapter, you will be able to:
- Discuss the importance of transfer documentation
- Define the importance of a structured approach to documentation

---

## 22.1 Introduction

Throughout this manual reference has been made to the need for communication to be both structured and concise. During a transfer the majority of communications are undertaken verbally, either face to face or by telephone (recording of telephone conference calls plays an increasingly important record in the transport process). It is important that the contents of key discussions are documented in the transport record and copies provided to both the referring and reciving hospitals for their notes.

In Chapter 21 clinical governance was discussed as a method to measure and deliver good quality care. Good documentation underpins this process and is essential for any subsequent case reviews or audit. All of the royal medical colleges and the Nursing and Midwifery Council (NMC) have issued statements about record keeping which are available to their members. Furthermore, it is worth noting that all NHS records are public records under the terms of the Public Records Act 1958, and therefore may be accessed by anyone with appropriate permissions.

## 22.2 Clinical notes

Clinical notes are a legal record and a log of events. It is vital that they record not only the interventions and decisions that are taken, but also the basic clinical information which prompted these actions. Alongside clinical care, biographical and logistical information and incidents should also be recorded. Clinicians' handwriting is notorious for its illegibility; it should be considered that there is little point in using the pen to communicate if no one else can decipher what was written.

If a fact or event is not documented then should you ever find yourself explaining your own actions in court the event is generally regarded as not to have happened. Furthermore, if an entry is illegible this not only represents a failure of communication but renders the entry inadmissible.

---

**CAUTION!**

Anything you do, or say, in the course of a patient's treatment, should be recorded in the clinical notes. If you do not clearly document what you have said or done, it will harm your defence, if you later rely on your memory.

---

As with all documentation, each entry in clinical notes should be dated, timed and signed. Furthermore, the author's name, General Medical Council (GMC) number if they are medical staff and status (e.g. consultant paediatrics) should be clearly appended (Figure 22.1). It is good practice to note the location of the child, for example, '18/12/2006 12:23 St Elsewhere PICU Smith J. (Paediatric Registrar) bleep 2341 (GMC No: 1234567)'. This may be especially useful should you need to refer to the notes of a retrieval to explain your actions subsequently.

---

*Neonatal, Adult and Paediatric Safe Transfer and Retrieval: A Practical Approach to Transfers*, First Edition.
Edited by Bernard Foëx, Peter-Marc Fortune and Cassie Lawn.
© 2019 John Wiley & Sons Ltd. Published 2019 by John Wiley & Sons Ltd.

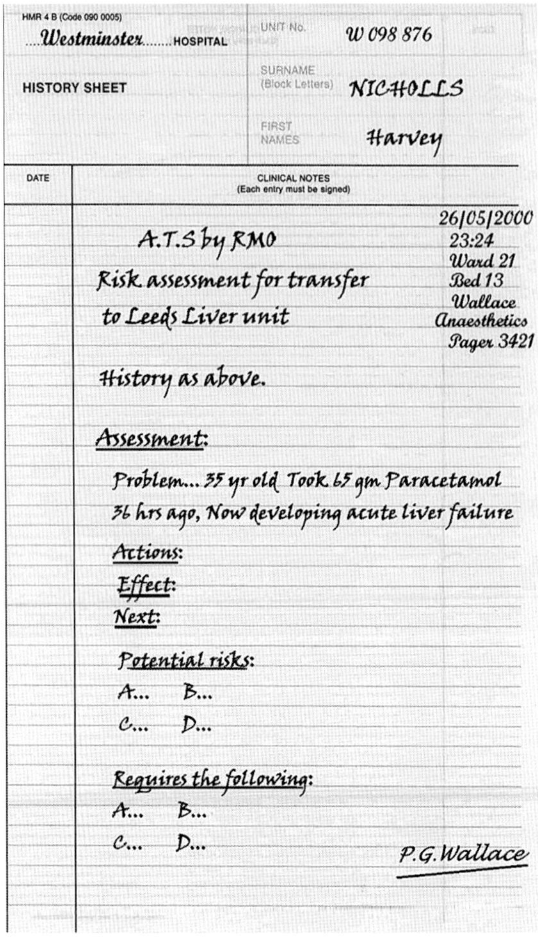
HMR 4 B (Code 090 0005)
....Westminster........HOSPITAL
HISTORY SHEET

UNIT No. W 098 876
SURNAME (Block Letters) NICHOLLS
FIRST NAMES Harvey

| DATE | CLINICAL NOTES (Each entry must be signed) |
| --- | --- |

A.T.S by RMO
Risk assessment for transfer to Leeds Liver unit

26/05/2000
23:24
Ward 21
Bed 13
Wallace
Anaesthetics
Pager 3421

History as above.

Assessment:

Problem... 35 yr old Took 65 gm Paracetamol 36 hrs ago, Now developing acute liver failure

Actions:
Effect:
Next:

Potential risks:
A... B...
C... D...

Requires the following:
A... B...
C... D...

P.G. Wallace

**Figure 22.1 Example of clinical notes**

It is vitally important to record the date and time when events occurred, as well as the time the entry was made. This is especially key when dealing with transfers, as the chronology of events and discussions may be crucial in an enquiry. If the pace of events and circumstances dictate that some entries must be made at a later time, then this must be made clear; the notes should state that it is a 'non-contemporaneous' or 'retrospective' entry. They should include the time of the event referred to as well as the time the entry was made.

As notes are written chronologically, there will inevitably be several sets of documentation covering:

- The referring hospital
- The transfer itself
- The receiving hospital

Where possible it is preferable that the documentation reads as one continuous record. The referring hospital clinical notes should clearly summarise:

- The patient's history
- The reasons for transfer
- Who has been involved in any discussions
- The assessments of the risks of transfer
- The consequent stabilisation procedures

This should end up with a statement such as: 'Patient transferred to St Elsewhere Hospital, Ward 101'.

A suggested framework for documenting pre-transfer care is:

- Date and time of referral
- Name of referring clinician
- Name of referring consultant
- Diagnosis
- Clinical status of patient
- Reason for transfer
- Actions agreed during referral process (and effect of these if any)
- Time of arrival and assessment of patient
- Status of patient on arrival
- Actions prior to transfer

Intensive care personnel and anaesthetists may be called to assess a child who is to be transferred to another hospital for care. The notes should clearly indicate the reason for the request. In such cases the approach should include an assessment of transfer risk and a logical evaluation leading to the conclusion about what staffing and equipment resources are required for this patient. An example is shown in Figure 22.2.

```
Patient's name:        DOB:
Problems:
1.
2.
3.
Request for transfer made by:
Reason for transfer:
Intended destination:
Summary clinical assessment:
Appropriate transfer? YES / NO
If Yes – Actions required before transfer / If No reason for declining
request:

Names and designations of transport team (if appropriate)
Transfer approved by ......................................................(Name of
consultant)
```

**Figure 22.2  Example of request for transfer**

## 22.3 Transfer forms

Some form of transfer documentation that provides a summary of care must be completed during and after the transfer.

Just as both hospitals will have a unique record number for each patient, the transport service will issue a unique record number for each ambulance journey – the transport number. This number should be recorded on the transfer form to facilitate audit and investigation of adverse incidents. Where a local ambulance service is used an incident number will also be produced and this should be recorded on the transport record.

Copies of the transfer form should be filed in the referring hospital's notes, the receiving hospital's notes and a central point for audit. Part of a sample transfer form is shown in Appendix D.

## 22.4  Summary

Effective oral and written communication is an essential part of the transfer process. All communication must be structured, clear and concise. Key oral communications should be recorded in the clinical notes.

The documentation of the events surrounding a transfer are important not only for clinical audit, but also for your own protection should litigation arise.

The last page of the referring hospital's notes, the transfer form and the first pages of the receiving hospital's notes should read as a seamless progression of events. The reader should be able to follow the thought processes that guided the chain of events bringing about the transfer of the critically ill person. The notes should also reflect the high standard of care and communication during this difficult time.

# PART 6
# Appendices

APPENDIX A

# Intensive care levels: classification of ICU patient dependency

This issue is classified by the paediatric intensive care unit (PICU) and neonatal intensive care unit (NICU) in slightly different ways.

- In the PICU the description is patient based but may be applied to describe a unit. For example, a level 1 critical care area, for children needing greater attention than can be provided on the ward, is generally classed as a high dependecy unit (HDU). Many district general hospitals (DGHs) will be able to provide level 2 care for a period of time without difficulty. However level 3 and 4 care is generally only delivered by specialised PICUs.
- In the NICU the description applies to the capabilities of the NICU itself. Similarly to above some DGHs will be able to provide level 1 care for a period of time but would only be expected to manage level 2 patients for short periods. These children are transferred to specialist NICU centres.
- For adults, levels of care are determined by the clinical needs of the patient (e.g. levels of organ support and/or monitoring) rather than the location where the care is delivered. Levels of care will determine the nurse : patient ratio. Typically level 0 and 1 care can be provided on acute hospital wards. HDUs will provide up to level 2 care, while level 3 care may be provided on intensive care units (ICUs), emergency department resuscitation rooms and theatre recovery areas.

*Neonatal, Adult and Paediatric Safe Transfer and Retrieval: A Practical Approach to Transfers*, First Edition.
Edited by Bernard Foëx, Peter-Marc Fortune and Cassie Lawn.

| Level of care | PICU | NICU | Adults |
|---|---|---|---|
| Level 0 | | | Patients needing less than 4 hourly observations (normal ward care). May have IV therapy |
| Level 1 | High dependency care requiring nurse : patient ratio 0.5:1 | Special care units (SCU) that provide special care but do not aim to provide continuing high dependency or intensive care. This category includes units with or without resident medical staff. Previously level 1 special care baby unit (SCBU) | Patients needing a minimum of 4 hourly observations. Typically includes patients who have stepped down from critical care to a ward; ward patients needing continuous oxygen therapy; patients with a tracheostomy or chest drain in place |
| Level 2 | A child requiring continuous nursing supervision who is usually intubated and ventilated. Also the unstable non intubated child (e.g. a child who has recently been extubated). Nurse : patient ratio 1:1 | Local neonatal units (LNUs) that provide high dependency care and some short term intensive care as agreed within their network. Previously level 2 SCBU | Patients needing single organ support (except basic respiratory and basic cardiovascular) or those needing preoperative optimisation, extended postoperative care, or stepping down from level 3 care. There should be a registered nurse : patient ratio of no less than 1:2 to deliver direct care |
| Level 3 | A child requiring intensive supervision at all times, who needs additional complex therapeutic procedures and nursing. For example, unstable ventilated children on vasoactive drugs, inotropic support or multiple organ failure. Level 2 children in a cubicle. Nurse : patient ratio 1.5:1 | NICUs that provide the whole range of medical neonatal care but not necessarily all specialist services such as neonatal surgery. Previously level 3 neonatal unit | Patients needing a minimum of two organ supports (except basic respiratory and basic cardiovascular) or advanced respiratory support alone (invasive mechanical ventilation or pressure support through a trans-laryngeal tracheal tube or tracheostomy tube, or continuous positive airway pressure through a trans-laryngeal tracheal tube). There should be a registered nurse : patient ratio of no less than 1:1 to deliver direct care |
| Level 4 | A child requiring the most intensive interventions such as level 3 patients nursed in a cubicle and children requiring renal replacement therapy. Nurse : patient ratio 2:1 | | |
| (Level 5) | This is a non-standardised definition for a child requiring intensive treatment modalities only available in quaternary centres. In practice this specifically refers to children requiring extracorporeal membrane oxygenation therapy. Nurse: patient ratio may be >2:1 | | |

# APPENDIX B
# Transfer quick reference

*Neonatal, Adult and Paediatric Safe Transfer and Retrieval: A Practical Approach to Transfers*, First Edition.
Edited by Bernard Foëx, Peter-Marc Fortune and Cassie Lawn.
© 2019 John Wiley & Sons Ltd. Published 2019 by John Wiley & Sons Ltd.

## Example of a transfer quick reference form

| **ASSESSMENT** |
| --- |
| What is the problem? (soundbite)<br>What is being done?<br>What effect is it having?<br>What is needed now? |

| **CONTROL** |
| --- |
| Identify team leader(s):<br>• Clinical<br>• Logistic<br>Identify tasks to be carried out<br>Allocate tasks to individuals/teams |

| **COMMUNICATION** | |
| --- | --- |
| Communication – what:<br>• Who you are<br>• Contact details<br>• What the problem is (soundbite)<br>• What you need from the listener<br>• What you have done<br>• Effect of these actions<br>• Summarise agreed plans | Communication – with who:<br>• Local team<br>• Transfer team<br>• Receiving team<br>• Ambulance control<br>• Family |

| **EVALUATION** |
| --- |
| Urgency of transfer<br>Appropriateness of transfer<br>Mode and speed of transport |

| **PREPARATION** |
| --- |
| Prepare:<br>• Patient<br>• Equipment<br>• Personnel<br>Package:<br>• Patient<br>• Equipment<br>Pre-departure checks |

| **TRANSPORTATION** |
| --- |
| Final check that destination is correct<br>Plan appropriate speed<br>Plan for adverse incidents<br>Load securely<br>Handover |

APPENDIX C
# Pre-departure checks

*Neonatal, Adult and Paediatric Safe Transfer and Retrieval: A Practical Approach to Transfers*, First Edition.
Edited by Bernard Foëx, Peter-Marc Fortune and Cassie Lawn.
© 2019 John Wiley & Sons Ltd. Published 2019 by John Wiley & Sons Ltd.

## Example of a pre-departure checks form

*Neonatal Transfer Service for Kent, Surrey & Sussex*

| Name: | | NHS no. | | DOB | |
|---|---|---|---|---|---|

| Discussion with parents |
|---|
| |
| Inpatient transfer of mum to receiving hospital arranged / being arranged |
| Parents offered transfer in ambulance:          Transfer Accepted          Transfer Refused |
| Parents making own way to receiving hospital |
| Parent information leaflet given |
| Directions / contact details for the receiving hospital given to parents |
| Contact number for parents MOBILE NO: |

### Pre-Departure Check list from Referring Hospital

| PATIENT | | DOCUMENTATION | | COMMUNICATION | | | | | |
|---|---|---|---|---|---|---|---|---|---|
| ETT Secure | | X-rays Checked | | Parents updated | | | | | |
| Name Bands x 2 | | X-rays taken or transmitted | | Religious Rites | | | | | |
| Drains / Lines Secure | | Drug Chart | | Transport Consultant updated | | | | | |
| Breast Milk | | Blood Spot– YES/NO/Unknown | | Receiving Unit Updated | | | | | |
| Clothing / Toys / photos | | BadgerNet Summary x 2 / Copy of Notes | | | | | | | |

### EVENTS DURING JOURNEY TO RECEIVING HOSPITAL

| | Time and Signature |
|---|---|
| | |

### PRE-DEPARTURE CHECK LIST AT RECEIVING HOSPITAL

| Prepacked Transport Bag | | Controlled Drugs | | | | | | | |
|---|---|---|---|---|---|---|---|---|---|
| Fridge Drugs | | Phones | | | | | | | |
| Copy of NTS Notes | | EBS Updated | | | | | | | |

| **LEAVING RECEIVING UNIT** | DAY_____/ _____/ 20 _____          TIME _____:_____ |
|---|---|

Name (Print) ..........................          Signature: ..........................

# APPENDIX D

# Generic forms: referral and transfer

*Neonatal, Adult and Paediatric Safe Transfer and Retrieval: A Practical Approach to Transfers*, First Edition.
Edited by Bernard Foëx, Peter-Marc Fortune and Cassie Lawn.

# NWTS REFERRAL FORM NWTS

North West & North Wales
Paediatric Transport Service

Referral Source: NWTS Direct / NWTS via _____
Please complete post-retrieval alterations to this form in red ink

| Referral Number: | | |
|---|---|---|

| Admin Name | Date Referral: | Time of Referral: | Check major trauma referral?' |
|---|---|---|---|
| NWTS Consultant | Date Transport agreed | Time transport agreed | NO / YES or Maybe - if yes or maybe<br>Bring NWTS cons & TTL in call immediately |

| Advice | Transfer | Bed request | HDU transfer | Neonatal transfer | Out of NWTS remit |
|---|---|---|---|---|---|

| Referring Hospital: | | Location: | |
|---|---|---|---|
| Referrer's Name: | | Grade and Speciality: | |
| Contact Number: | Direct Line<br>Mobile: | Switchboard<br>Bleep Number: | |
| Referring Consultant: | Name: | Contact number: | Referring Consultant?<br>Present / Aware / Unaware |

**Child's name:** First name    Surname

DOB:    Age:

Home Address:    Gestation: /40

Corrected Age: (if less than 2 yrs)

Postcode

NHS No:    Sex:    Weight:

Child known to PICU? If yes: RMCH    AHCH    OTHER ................

Does this child have a ReSPECT Form or Life Plan? Yes / No    Is this child known to NWTS? Yes / No

Speciality consultant in conferenced call?
Name: .........................................
Speciality: ..............Hospital: ...........

| Ambulance booking no. | |
|---|---|
| PICANet ID Number | |
| Transfer Form? | Yes / No |
| Blue Light Form? | Yes / No |
| Safeguarding Form? | Yes / No |
| Observation printout photocopied & in notes | Yes / not applicable |
| Form scanned (NWTS) | Yes / No |
| Admin: check all tasks complete once case closed | Signature |
| NWTS transferred on: | Date |

**BEFORE CLOSING CASE PLEASE CHECK FOLLOWING:**

| Follow up min 24 hours done | Yes / No |
|---|---|
| Notes complete & date/signed? | Yes / No |
| Prescription/fluid section? | Complete: Yes / No / NA |
| Does this patient have a difficult airway? YES / NO | Check all notes complete & flagged on database |
| Incident ? No / Yes<br>YES attach incident form (s) | Form Number: |
| Excellence Report ?<br>No / Yes | Form submitted: Yes / No<br>Not applicable |
| Flight transfer—considered?<br>No / Yes—check reasons for decline recorded | For ALL flight transfers please use flight transfer form |
| Database: name to confirm | Dr    Nurse |
| Date Closed / Cons signature | |

NWTS Referral number: 08000 84 83 82  NWTS Mobile 1: 07825 231737  Mobile 2: 07825 231822  Mobile 3: 07825 231 768  Admin mobile: 07825 231753
RMCH Senior Nurse: 0161-701-8022  RMCH Bed Consultant: 0161-701-8224  AHCH Number: 0151 252 5242/41  Security Birchwood: 01925 858853
1
NWTS Referral Form version 3.1 11.12.18    Not to be reviewed till April 2019

Name:

Number:        DOB:

---

**Provisional Diagnosis:**

---

## Clinical Details at time of referral:

| Date & time of admission to referring hospital: | Time of injury or ingestion: | Allergies: |
|---|---|---|
| NWTS information taken by (name): | NWTS consultant in call:  Yes / No  - if no why?<br><br>Paediatric consultant in call: Yes / No—if no why?<br><br>TTL in the call: Yes / No / NA    - If NO why? | |

TRIAGE QUESTIONS:  Is the child in cardiac arrest?  Yes / No        Is the child in extremis?  Yes / No

| **Anaesthetic Assessment Done?** | **YES / NO / AWAITED** | |
|---|---|---|
| **Anaesthetist Name & Grade:** | **Assessment Time:** | |
| **Mat. Pertussis vaccination in pregnancy (pts < 6/12)?** | YES / NO / N/A | **Immunisations up to date?** YES / NO |

# Observations and Investigations at time of referral

Name:

Number:

## AIRWAY

| Own | ☐ | Trache? | ☐ | LTV | ☐ |
|---|---|---|---|---|---|

| Clear / Compromised | Size / length / cuff | Settings / FiO₂ / Vent |
|---|---|---|

| I&V / Adjuncts | | |
|---|---|---|

## BREATHING

| RR | ET CO₂ | SpO₂ | FiO₂ |
|---|---|---|---|

↑WOB? No / Yes:   Intercostal / Subcostal recession

Tracheal tug / Nasal flaring / Grunting / Head bobbing

Gastric tube? No / Yes    Oral / Nasal / Gastrostomy / Other

High Flow Humid. O₂? No / Yes   Flow: L/min

NIV? No / Yes   CPAP / BiPAP?
Flow: L/min          Pressures:          Back-up rate (BiPAP):

Invasive Vent: Yes / No    Mode:      TV (ml/kg):
Pressures:           Ti:          Rate:

| CXR | Chest Exam: |
|---|---|

## Circulation

| HR | BP | CRT: C | CRT: P |
|---|---|---|---|
| IO | Peripheral venous | Central venous | Arterial |
| Fluid Bolus (ml/kg) | Crystalloid | Colloid | Blood |

| Maintenance | | | |
|---|---|---|---|

| Inotropes | | **Murmur?** | |
|---|---|---|---|
| **PU in last 6-12 hrs?** | | **Palpable Liver?** | **Femoral Pulses?** |

## Disability

| GCS   /15 | E | V | M | A  V  P  U |
|---|---|---|---|---|
| CT Head: | Yes / No | | Sedation | |
| Seizures: | Yes / No | | Paralysis | |
| Pupils | Left | Right | 2.7% saline | Mannitol |

## Abdomen

| Abdomen distended & tense? Yes / No | Imaging? |
|---|---|
| Vomiting bile? Yes / No | |

## Sepsis 6 Pathway triggered? Yes / No   Check complete?

| High flow O2? | IV / IO fluid bolus? |
|---|---|
| IV / IO access + bloods sent? | Senior Paeds review? |
| IV antimicrobials given? | Inotropes considered? |

## Blood Gas Results

| | | | | |
|---|---|---|---|---|
| Date/Time | | | | |
| FiO₂ | | | | |
| A / C / V | | | | |
| pH | | | | |
| pCO₂ | | | | |
| pO₂ | | | | |
| HCO₃ | | | | |
| BXS | | | | |
| Lactate | | | | |
| Glucose | | | | |
| Other | | | | |

## Laboratory Results

| | | | |
|---|---|---|---|
| Date / Time | | | |
| Hb | | | |
| WCC/Neuts /Lymphs | | | |
| Platelets | | | |
| PT/INR | | | |
| APTT / APTT ratio | | | |
| Fibrinogen | | | |
| D Dimer | | | |
| Na | | | |
| K | | | |
| Urea | | | |
| Creatinine | | | |
| CRP | | | |
| Calcium | | | |
| Magnesium | | | |
| Ammonia | | | |
| Bilirubin / Albumin | | | |
| ALT / AST | | | |
| ALP / GGT | | | |
| Toxicology sent? | | | |

## SEPSIS

| Temp: | | |
|---|---|---|
| **Cultures:** Blood / Urine / PCR / CSF / Sputum / NPA (viral) | | |
| **Which antimicrobial (s) given** If meningitis (> 3 mnths) check dexamethasone (0.15 mg/kg) given? | | |
| **Any known resistance?** | | |

Name:

Number:          DOB:

## Advice Given

### Please sign, date and time all entries

Name of referring clinician that advice was passed to:

Advice agreed with referrer?

1.

| Has intubation been advised? | Y / N |
| --- | --- |
| Advised to use an intubation check list & consider plan A, B, C (intubation guideline)? | Y / N |

2.

| Advised to draw up bolus fluid & resus dose adrenaline diluted in 10-20 mls? | Y / N |
| --- | --- |

3.

4.

5.

6.

| Additional Blood Gas Results | |
| --- | --- |
| Time Taken | |
| Art/Cap/Ven | |
| pH | |
| $pCO_2$ | |
| $pO_2$ | |
| $HCO_3$ | |
| BXS | |
| Lactate | |
| Glucose | |
| Na | |
| K | |
| iCa | |
| Hb | |

**Follow-up: include clinical observations & blood gas / other blood results (actual numbers)**

**Please sign, date and time all entries**

| Additional Blood Gas Results | | | |
|---|---|---|---|
| Time Taken | | | |
| Art/Cap/Ven | | | |
| pH | | | |
| pCO2 | | | |
| pO2 | | | |
| HCO3 | | | |
| BXS | | | |
| Lactate | | | |
| Glucose | | | |
| Na | | | |
| K | | | |
| iCa | | | |
| Hb | | | |

NWTS Referral Form version 3.1 11.12.18          Not to be reviewed till April 2019

Name:

Number:          DOB:

---

**Follow-up: include clinical observations & blood gas / other blood results (actual numbers)**

**Please sign, date and time all entries**

| Additional Blood Gas Results | | |
|---|---|---|
| Time Taken | | |
| Art/Cap/Ven | | |
| pH | | |
| pCO2 | | |
| pO2 | | |
| HCO3 | | |
| BXS | | |
| Lactate | | |
| Glucose | | |
| Na | | |
| K | | |
| iCa | | |
| Hb | | |

Name:

Number:          DOB:

**Follow-up: include clinical observations & blood gas / other blood results (actual numbers)**

**Please sign, date and time all entries**

| Additional Blood Gas Results | | |
|---|---|---|
| Time Taken | | |
| Art/Cap/Ven | | |
| pH | | |
| pCO2 | | |
| pO2 | | |
| HCO3 | | |
| BXS | | |
| Lactate | | |
| Glucose | | |
| Na | | |
| K | | |
| iCa | | |
| Hb | | |

NWTS Referral Form version 3.1 11.12.18          Not to be reviewed till April 2019

| PICANet Data—Referral | Name: |
| --- | --- |
| | Number:        DOB: |

## Complete for ALL patients referred to NWTS

| Referring Unit: | | | | Referring Speciality: | | | |
| --- | --- | --- | --- | --- | --- | --- | --- |

| **Grade of Referring Doctor or Nurse** | Consultant/ Ass Specialist | ST4-8 | ST1-3 | F1/F2 | GP | ANP | Nurse | Unknown |
| --- | --- | --- | --- | --- | --- | --- | --- | --- |

| Was patient receiving invasive ventilation (via ETT, LMA or tracheostomy at time referral accepted? | Yes | No—not indicated | No—advised to intubate | Unknown |
| --- | --- | --- | --- | --- |

| **Referral Outcome** | **Accepted— for NWTS transfer** | **Refused— no team** | **Refused—time critical** | **Refused—out of NWTS remit** | **Transfer / bed request from neonatal team** |
| --- | --- | --- | --- | --- | --- |
| **Bed request from OOR transport team**<br><br>KIDS / Embrace / Nectar / WATCh / CATS / STRS / SORT / COMET | **Advice ONLY:** indicate max support<br><br>HFHO$_2$ / NIV / I&V for seizures & extubated locally / inotropes / Other | **Comments incl. reason NWTS refused** | | | |

| **Admission outcome** | | PICU | NICU | AICU—DGH | HDU—DGH | HDU—tertiary | Ward—DGH | Ward—tertiary | Hospice / Home |
| --- | --- | --- | --- | --- | --- | --- | --- | --- | --- |
| Unit 1: | Time | PICM consultant | | Accepted— NWTS request | | Refused—no staffed bed | | Refused—out of scope of care | Bed request from OOR team—accepted |
| Unit 2: | Time | PICM Consultant | | Accepted— NWTS request | | Refused—no staffed bed | | Refused—out of scope of care | Bed request from OOR team—accepted |
| Unit 3: | Time | PICM Consultant | | Accepted— NWTS request | | Refused—no staffed bed | | Refused—out of scope of care | |
| Unit 4: | Time | PICM Consultant | | Accepted— NWTS request | | Refused—no staffed bed | | Refused—out of scope of care | |
| Unit 5: | Time | PICM Consultant | | Accepted— NWTS request | | Refused—no staffed bed | | Refused—out of scope of care | |
| Unit 6: | Time | PICM Consultant | | Accepted— NWTS request | | Refused—no staffed bed | | Refused—out of scope of care | |

| **Transport team?** | NWTS | NWTS/PIC extra: specify | Neonatal team: specify | DGH?<br><br>Anaes / Paed | Other PIC transport team:<br>KIDS / Embrace / Nectar / WATCh / CATS / STRS / SORT / COMET |
| --- | --- | --- | --- | --- | --- |

| **Referral Category** | Respiratory | Cardiac | ECMO | Sepsis | Poisoning |
| --- | --- | --- | --- | --- | --- |
| Neurology | Metabolic | Renal | Liver | Haem / Onc | Endocrine |
| Burns | Surgical Neonate | General Surgical | ENT | Neurosurgery | Trauma |
| Palliative Care | PICU back transfer | Other | | | |

| **PICANet data verified by:** | | **PICANet Data entered by:** | |
| --- | --- | --- | --- |

**Comments:** if referral outcome = advice only, please include any excellence or adverse incidents here

Please ensure that you take both referral and transfer form with you

**North West & North Wales
Paediatric Transport Service**

| Referral Number |
| --- |

# NWTS TRANSFER FORM

| Name: | | DOB: | Age: |
| --- | --- | --- | --- |
| NHS Number: | | | |
| Collection Area: | | Sex: | Weight: |
| Destination Unit: | | Date transfer agreed | Time transfer agreed |

| NWTS Umbrella Safety check: | | | Estimated journey time: | |
| --- | --- | --- | --- | --- |
| Team composition discussed / agreed | YES/NO | | **Flight considered (if > 120 mins)? Yes / No** | |
| RISK SCORE (record result) If > 4 reduce risk eg exchange/add team member/driver; delay transfer; change route (document actions) | | | **Service? TCAA / EMTRS / Other** Indicate why refused | |
| | | | Service unavailable (specify) | Pt not suitable for flight eg can't lie flat (specify) |
| Consultant on transfer—if Yes why? | YES/NO | | Weather | Night Flight |
| Trainee or nurse support / supervision; Patient acuity Consultant on transport doctor shift Additional team / Logistics / Consultant choice / Other (state): | | | Other: | |
| | | | Sea Air Rescue (SAR) team considered if poor weather or night flight required? Yes / No / Refusal (state reason) | |

| TRANSPORT TIMES | Base to Collecting Unit | Patient Journey | Destination unit to Base |
| --- | --- | --- | --- |
| Mode of transport Please clarify | NWTS Ambulance Other? | NWTS Ambulance Other? | NWTS Ambulance Other? |
| Departing Times: | Base: | Collection Unit: | Destination: |
| Ambulance Category | GREEN AMBER **RED** | GREEN AMBER **RED** | GREEN AMBER **RED** |
| Arrival Times: | Collection Unit: | Destination Unit: | Base: |
| Blue lights or siren used | YES / NO | YES / NO | YES / NO |
| Organisational delay Which journey affected? | No / Yes—cause? Team out Staffing Vehicle Details: | | Awaiting PICU bed Document time ready to leave: |
| Vehicle Incident | None / Yes— Accident / Breakdown Please complete incident form (full details) | | |
| 2nd NWTS team | Departure from base: Time of handover (between NWTS teams): | | |

| Checklist as leaving NWTS Base | | | | Transport Team—specify Day / Night / 12-12 / Other | |
| --- | --- | --- | --- | --- | --- |
| Mobile Phone | | Referral & Transfer Form | | **Name (Team leader first)** | **Grade:** |
| CMAC, Sonosite + iSTAT | | Crash Call & Document Folder | | | |
| Gas Status Checked & Gas Calculation done? | | Airway Kit, Bagging Circuit & AMBU Bag | | | |
| Fridge Drug Pack | | Central Line | | | |
| Monitor Bag | | Appropriate Vent Circuit | | | |
| If NIV check approp mask for older child? | | NWAS bag & straps if using NWAS | | | |

# Name of Doctor, grade and specialty delivering handover:

Most senior member present at collecting unit:

| Assessment made by NWTS Team | Initial assessment time: | Clinical examination / assessment: | Pre-departure status time: |
|---|---|---|---|
| Intubated: Yes/No<br><br>If no: any airway support required?  Yes / No | ETT / Trache:<br><br>Oral / Nasal / Trache<br><br>Cuffed / Uncuffed<br><br>Size:          Length: | ETT position checked on CXR: Yes / No<br><br>NGT position checked on CXR? Yes / No<br><br>pH testing?  Yes / No<br><br>**Document  CXR findings:** | Any changes made to ETT or NGT position?<br><br>Sputum sample  Y / N<br><br>Manual decompression Y / N |
| Ventilation Mode | HFHO$_2$ / Non-Invasive / Invasive | | HFHO$_2$ / Non-Invasive / Invasive |
| FiO$_2$ | | **Respiratory examination:** | |
| SpO$_2$ | | | |
| Respiratory Rate | | | |
| ET CO$_2$ | | | |
| PIP / PEEP / Flow | | | |
| Mean Airway Press | | | |
| Ti / TV | | | |
| Blood Gas? | | | |
| Nitric Oxide (ppm) | | | |
| Heart Rate | | HS: | |
| BP Sys/Dia (Mean) | | | |
| Cap Refill Time | | Peripheral Pulses? | |
| CPR In progress | Yes/No | Please indicate where | Yes/No |
| Inotropes | | palpable | |
| Resus Fluid Given | | | |
| Passed Urine? | | On ALL patients—complete diagram | |
| Temperature | | Any organomegaly?  No / Yes | |
| NGT present? Y / N | Aspirated? Y / N | Masses? Scars? | NGT aspirated? Y / N |
| Blood Sugar | | | |
| Maintenance fluid? | | | |
| GCS | | | |
| PEARL | Yes/No | Other marks / rashes? | Yes/No |
| Left / Right Size | R          L | | R          L |
| Sedation Analgesia Paralysis | | Tone / Power / Posture: Normal or abnormal<br><br>Describe if abnormal: | |
| Mannitol/2.7%Saline ?  Y / N | | Anterior Fontanelle: sunken / normal / bulging | Y / N |

10

## NWTS Prescription Chart

**ALL INFUSIONS OR DRUGS GIVEN WHILST NWTS PRESENT MUST BE PRESCRIBED. KEEP A COPY OF REFERRING UNITS' PRESCRIPTION & FLUID CHART IN NWTS RECORDS**

Name:

Number:          DOB:

| Patient's Weight | Copy of crash call?  YES / NO |
|---|---|

**ALLERGIES:**

| INFUSION DRUGS (Pump Name) | PRESCRIBER'S SIGNATURE | DOSE RANGE | RATE RANGE (mls/hour) | CONCENTRATION | CHECKED BY / ADMIN BY | PUMP NAME | START TIME |
|---|---|---|---|---|---|---|---|
| MORPHINE | | 10–40 micrograms/ kg/hr | | **mg  in 50ml** (1mg/kg in 50mls) | | | |
| FENTANYL | | 1–4 micrograms/ kg/hr | | **micrograms in 50 ml** (50 micrograms/kg in 50mls) | | | |
| MIDAZOLAM | | 60–240 micrograms/kg/hr | | **mg in 50ml** (3mg/kg in 50mls) | | | |
| DOPAMINE | | 5–20 micrograms/kg/min | | **mg in 50ml** (15mg/kg in 50mls) | | | |
| ADRENALINE | | 0.1–1 micrograms/kg/min | | **mg in 50ml** (0.3mg/kg in 50mls) | | | |
| | | | | | | | |
| | | | | | | | |
| HEPARIN | | Arterial Line | **1ml/hr** | **500 units in 500mls** **0.9% Saline** | | | |
| MAINTENANCE FLUID (include type) | | | | Type of fluid: | | | |

| Bolus Drug/Fluid | Dose | Route | Total Volume | Over (duration) | Prescriber's Signature | Check / Admin | Time Administered |
|---|---|---|---|---|---|---|---|
| ROCURONIUM 1mg/kg | mg | | | STAT | | | |
| ROCURONIUM 1mg/kg | mg | | | STAT | | | |
| | | | | | | | |
| | | | | | | | |
| | | | | | | | |
| | | | | | | | |
| | | | | | | | |
| | | | | | | | |
| | | | | | | | |
| | | | | | | | |
| | | | | | | | |
| | | | | | | | |
| | | | | | | | |

NWTS Transfer Form version 3.0 28.03.18   Not to be reviewed till October 2018

Name:

## Patient Observations

| | Time | | | | | | | | | | | |
|---|---|---|---|---|---|---|---|---|---|---|---|---|
| **Temperature, Site:** | | | | | | | | | | | | |

| | | |
|---|---|---|
| | **200** | |
| **HR - 0** | **190** | |
| **BP - ^** | **180** | |
| **MAP- x** | **170** | |
| **RR - +** | **160** | |
| **CVP - Δ** | **150** | |
| | **140** | |
| Cooling/warming measures used: | **130** | |
| | **120** | |
| Baby Pod | | |
| Transwarmer | **110** | |
| Inditherm | **100** | |
| Medi Wrap | **90** | |
| Bubble Wrap | **80** | |
| Blankets | **70** | |
| Hat | **60** | |
| Ice Packs | **50** | |
| Other | **40** | |
| | **30** | |
| | **20** | |
| | **10** | |
| **Mean BP** | | |

| | | |
|---|---|---|
| **Ventilation** | **Mode** | |
| **Vent name:** | **FiO$_2$** | |
| | **SpO$_2$** | |
| | **Rate** | |
| | **PIP/PEEP** | |
| | **MAP** | |
| | **TV** | |
| | **ET CO$_2$** | |
| **Nitric** | **PPM** | |

| | |
|---|---|
| **Pupil Size/Reaction R** | |
| **Pupil Size/Reaction L** | |

| Rate / Press | |
|---|---|
| Morphine/Fentanyl - mcg/kg/hr | |
| Midazolam—mcg/kg/hr | |
| Maintenance—ml/hr | |
| | |
| | |
| | |

12

## INTUBATION—FOR EVERY PATIENT (not just those intubated by NWTS team)

| Time of Intubation | | Before NWTS arrived?  Yes / No |
|---|---|---|
| Intubated by: (speciality / grade) | Anaes / Paeds / Neo / PICM / NWTS      ST4-8 / ANP / Cons / Other | |
| Indication | Unable to maintain airway / Respiratory Failure / Airway obstruction risk / Increased WOB / Risk or actual apnoea / Reduced level of consciousness / Cardiac arrest / Sepsis / Metabolic demand / Other: | |
| Method of induction: | Rapid Sequence Induction (RSI) / Modified RSI / Elective IV induction / Inhalation / None / Other: | |
| Induction agents and dose used  Muscle relaxant and dose used | | |
| Laryngoscopy grade: | I (Easy) / II / III / IV | **NUMBER OF ATTEMPTS** |
| Did laryngoscopy grade improve with repositioning / cricoid pressure? Yes/ No | | |
| **NWTS CMAC USED?** | No / Yes  (place sticker here) | |
| Any airway adjuncts used? | Guedel / Bougie / LMA / Cricoid Pressure / None / Other:   Videolaryngoscope (not NWTS): Yes / No | |
| Any complications/difficulties? | Difficult airway / Hypotension / Hypoxia / Bradycardia / Pneumothorax / Cardiac Arrest / None / Other: | |
| Location | A&E / Paeds Ward / PHDU / Theatre/Recovery / NICU / Other: | |

## CENTRAL LINE—for every patient—not just those inserted by NWTS

| Indication | Pressure Monitoring / Blood sampling / Drugs / Access / Transfusion / Other: | | |
|---|---|---|---|
| Parents informed | Yes / No | Insertion site | Right or Left |
| Catheter type, size, length & no. lumens | | | |
| Number of attempts | State where/why failed: | | |
| Strict asepsis (indicate) | Hat / mask / gown / gloves / sterile drape / 2% Chloraprep / Biopatch / Sterile dressing | | |
| Ultrasound used | Yes / No | Sterile Sheath and gel | Yes / No |
| Guide wire removed | Yes | Blood Gas Checked | Yes / No |
| Tip Confirmed on CXR | Yes / No / Not applicable | Line transduced | Yes / No |
| Any complications? | None / Pneumothorax / Haemorrhage / Malposition / Arterial puncture / Other: | | |
| Line inserted by:  Name, Grade, Speciality: | | | |

## ARTERIAL LINE—for every patient—not just those inserted by NWTS

| Indication | Pressure Monitoring / Blood sampling / Other: | |
|---|---|---|
| Insertion site : | Right or Left | Parents informed?  Yes / No |
| No of attempts & state where/why failed: | | Catheter type, size, length |
| Strict asepsis (indicate) | Hat / mask / gown / gloves / sterile drape / 2% Chloraprep / Biopatch / Sterile dressing | |
| Ultrasound used | Yes / No | Sterile Sheath and gel   Yes / No |
| Guide wire removed | Yes | Blood Gas Checked   Yes / No |
| Any complications? | No / Yes—specify: | |
| Line Inserted by: Name, Grade, Speciality | | |

Name:

Number:　　　　DOB:

| Intervention + indication | ie Urinary catheter, chest drain, other | | | |
|---|---|---|---|---|
| **Parents informed** | Yes / No | **Insertion site** | | Right or Left |
| **Size** | | | | |
| **Number of attempts** | State where/why failed: | | | |
| **Strict asepsis (indicate)** | hat / mask / sterile drape / gown / gloves / 2% Chloraprep or Saline (for cleaning) | | | |
| **Confirm placement by** | | | | |
| **Any complications?** | No / Yes: specify: | | | |
| **Intervention by: Name, Grade, Speciality:** | | | | |

| | Date and Time Taken & indicate which gas used for PIMS score: | | | | | | | | |
|---|---|---|---|---|---|---|---|---|---|
| **Gases** | Arterial/Venous/Capillary: | | | | | | | | |
| | $FiO_2$ | | | | | | | | |
| | pH | | | | | | | | |
| | $pCO_2$ kPa | | | | | | | | |
| | $pO_2$ kPa | | | | | | | | |
| | $HCO_3$ mmol/l | | | | | | | | |
| | BE mmol/l | | | | | | | | |
| | Lactate | | | | | | | | |
| | Met Hb | | | | | | | | |
| | Oxygenation Index (OI) | | | | | | | | |
| | **OI = $FiO_2$ (%) x MAP (mmHg) x 100/$PaO_2$ (mmHg)    mmHg = kPa x 7.5** | | | | | | | | |
| **Labs** | Na+ mmol/l | | | | | | | | |
| | K+ mmol/l | | | | | | | | |
| | Ca++ mmol/l | | | | | | | | |
| | Blood Glucose | | | | | | | | |
| | Hb | | | | | | | | |
| | Chloride mmol/l | | | | | | | | |
| | $SpO_2$ | | | | | | | | |
| | AMMONIA | | | | | | | | |

| Interventions | By DGH | By NWTS | Interventions | By DGH | By NWTS |
|---|---|---|---|---|---|
| Primary Intubation | | | Primary intraosseous access | | |
| Re-intubation | | | Additional intraosseous access | | |
| Other Airway | | | Chest Drain Insertion | | |
| Non-invasive ventilation | | | Naso/Orogastric Tube | | |
| High flow humidified $O_2$ | | | Urinary Catheter | | |
| Primary Central venous access | | | Suction & saline lavage | | |
| Arterial access | | | Additional intervention (s) | | |
| Inotrope/Vasopressor infusion | | | | | |
| Prostaglandin Infusion | | | Total Fluid Resus Given (mls/kg) | | |
| Peripheral venous line (nos.) | | | | | |

Name:

Number:          DOB:

**NWTS clinical summary**

**Include probable diagnosis, patient history, current problems & results of any treatment / interventions**

NWTS Transfer Form version 3.0 28.03.18   Not to be reviewed till October 2018

**NWTS clinical summary (continued)**

16

| **Family** | Parents / Guardian Names | Contact Numbers | Parents in Ambulance Y/N  1 or 2?<br>Yes – other family member<br>No – Parent not present<br>No – Parent not permitted<br>No – Parent declined to accompany<br>If no, how did parent travel:<br>Own car / Taxi / Police / Flight /<br>Ferry / Train / Other: |
|---|---|---|---|
| Information Leaflet given Yes / No<br><br>Consent required? Y / N          Consent taken by: | | | Interpreter required  Yes / No<br><br>Parents language: |
| Parents spoken to by:<br><br>Information given: | | | Family History: |

| GENERAL INFORMATION TO BE COMPLETED FOR ALL PATIENTS | YES | NO |
|---|---|---|
| Does the family have a social worker or are they known to social care? | | |
| Name:                    Area:                    Contact number: | | |
| Social worker informed of this admission? | | |
| Who has parental responsibility? | | |
| Is the patient a 'child in need' (ie child requires extra help from professionals to achieve or maintain health and/or development)? | | |
| Is the patient a 'looked after child' (eg foster care or placed with parents with social services input)? | | |
| Any previous or current safeguarding concerns? | | |
| Any history, injury or incident raising safeguarding concerns eg inconsistent history, OOHCA? | | |
| **If yes to any of above please complete separate NWTS safeguarding form** | | |

**Please document any marks/Injuries (document size, colour of any marks/injuries) & position lines/tubes**

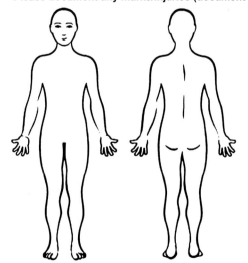

| Type of fluid | Fluid output |
|---|---|
| Urine (mls) | |
| Bowels | |
| Vomit / NG (mls) | |

| |
|---|
| Immunisations up to date? Yes   /   No |
| Maternal pertussis vaccination (< 6/12)?  Yes  / No |

Name:

Number:            DOB:

| Communication Check BEFORE leaving referring unit (NOT to be done in the ambulance) | |
|---|---|
| Pre-departure Clinical Assessment Done | Y/N |
| NWTS Consultant informed & journey/management plan agreed | Y/N |
| Receiving Consultant informed of departure and ETA  Name: | Y/N |
| Receiving Senior Nurse informed of departure & ETA  Name: | Y/N |
| Is a cubicle required? | Y/N |
| Notes, recent clinic letter, drug / fluids /observation charts + any ECGs or rhythm strips copied | Y/N |
| Any radiology eg CXR, CT scans sent via PACS | Y/N |
| Name band or Mepitac label on patient | Y/N |

| Equipment Checklist as leaving referring unit | |
|---|---|
| Mobile Phone +  Document Folder | Y/N |
| ISTAT | Y/N |
| CMAC | Y/N |
| Sonosite | Y/N |
| Check sufficient gas quantity for journey (do gas calculation if on HFHO$_2$—oxygen only) | Y/N |
| Airway kit, bagging circuit & AMBU Bag ready | Y/N |
| Emergency Drugs/Fluids + drug line available | Y/N |
| PIM Score (page 20) complete | Y/N |
| Parents updated and aware of plan. | Y/N |

| If Patient died before transfer  - checklist | |
|---|---|
| 'When a child dies' NWTS booklet given to family | Y/N |
| SUDC Paediatrician informed | Y/N |
| Please complete separate checklist & attach to form | |

| SUMMARY: on-going problems & any transfer events etc | |
|---|---|
| Date + time | |
| | |
| | |
| | |
| | |
| | |
| | |
| | |
| | |
| | |

| | |
|---|---|
| Doctor Signature/print name: | Nurse Signature/print name: |
| Care handed over to (medic/ANP: name/grade): | Care handed over to (Nurse: name/grade): |

NWTS Transfer Form version 3.0 28.03.18   Not to be reviewed till October 2018

Name:

Number:                    DOB:

| Any blood products transported ? | Yes / No | | Timing of any loading doses or drugs that will continue that have started at DGH? |
|---|---|---|---|
| Any blood products not used handed over to transfusion? | Yes / No | | E.g. antimicrobials (start date), potassium, magnesium, calcium, anticonvulsants, paracetamol |
| If not— document why? | | | **Drug Name** · **Time last dose** |

| **Pre-departure Checklist as leaving Receiving Unit** | |
|---|---|
| Both forms copied & copy left at receiving unit | Y/N |
| Mobile Phone | Y/N |
| Document Folder + original NWTS form | Y/N |
| Any additional NWTS notes | Y/N |
| Trolley & Kit Cleaned | Y/N |
| Drugs Disposed of | Y/N |

| **24 hours post transfer to PICU** | |
|---|---|
| **Did Child survive?  YES / NO** | |
| If no please check following................ | |
| Was organ donation considered | Yes / No |
| Has coroner agreed that death certificate can be issued? | Yes / No |
| NWTS cons. completed pt summary & filed in notes | Yes / No |
| Patient summary sent to relevant team | Yes / No |

| Date | **POST TRANSFER OUTCOME**—include ventilation details (& time of extubation), any inotropes, additional therapies (CVVH / ECMO etc), final culture results, final diagnosis, cause of death (if known) etc |
|---|---|
| | |

NWTS Transfer Form version 3.0 28.03.18   Not to be reviewed till October 2018

Name:

Number:          DOB:

## PIM2/PIM3 Information

Complete for all patients that a NWTS team is sent to even if transfer is not undertaken

| Planned admission to PICU? | Y | N |
|---|---|---|

| **Main Reason for Admission** | | | |
|---|---|---|---|
| Asthma | Bronchiolitis | Croup | Obstructive Sleep Apnoea |
| Recovery from surgery : | | | |
| Bypass cardiac procedure | Non-bypass cardiac procedure | Elective Liver transplant | Other procedure |
| Diabetic Ketoacidosis | Seizure Disorder | Other (none of the above) | |

| Observations recorded in 1st hr NWTS physical contact | |
|---|---|
| Systolic Blood Pressure | mmHg |
| Blood Gas Measured | Yes/No  A / V /C |
| Arterial PaO$_2$ | (kPa/mmHg) |
| FiO$_2$ at time of sample | |
| Intubated at time of sample? | Yes or No |
| Head box at time of sample? | Yes or No |
| Base Excess | mmol/l |
| Lactate | mmol/l |
| Mechanical Ventilation | Yes or No |
| CPAP | Yes or No |
| Pupil Reaction | Fixed and Dilated / Other / Unknown |

| Is information available to assess past medical history?   Yes   /   No       (circle applicable) | | | |
|---|---|---|---|
| Cardiac arrest before NWTS arrived | Cardiac arrest OUT of hospital | Cardiomyopathy or myocarditis | Hypoplastic Left Heart Syndrome |
| Severe Combined Immune Deficiency | Leukaemia or Lymphoma after first induction | Liver Failure main reason for ICU admission | Acute NEC main reason for ICU admission |
| Spontaneous Cerebral Haemorrhage | Neurodegenerative disorder | Human Immunodeficiency Virus (HIV) | Bone Marrow transplant recipient |

| Critical Incidents while Transport Team in Attendance   YES   /   NO | | |
|---|---|---|
| Accidental extubation | Loss of all IV Access | **Other:** |
| Required intubation in transit | Cardiac Arrest | Out of region transfer<br>HDU level transfer |
| Complete ventilator failure | Medication administration error | Prescribing error<br>Other (specify below) |
| Loss of medical gas supply | Equipment failure/incompatibility impacting on patient care | |

**EQUIPMENT (any failure): complete medical devices form & arrange for the equipment to be checked by MEAM at MFT**

Signed_____          Date_____

Other, Specify:

| NWTS Consultant aware: Yes / No | NWTS senior nurse aware: Yes / No | |
|---|---|---|

**Incident form completed: Yes / No** NB please print out 2 copies of incident form—one stays with NWTS form + hand one to admin

| Transport Outcome: | Patient Transported | Not Transported | | | Patient died | | |
|---|---|---|---|---|---|---|---|
| | Unplanned / Planned | Condition Improved | Condition deteriorated | Other reason | Before NWTS arrived | NWTS present | During transit |
| **Destination:** | RMCH/AHCH/Stoke/Other | PICU | PHDU | AICU | Ward/ED/Theatre | NICU | Home/Hospice |

# APPENDIX E
# Glossary

**AC**   Alternating current

**Afterload**   The pressure the ventricles must pump against to eject blood

**ALS** (advanced life support)   A structured system for the management of cardiac arrests designed in the USA in the 1970s. The Advanced Life Support Course (ALS) refers to the nationally recognised provider programme run by the UK Resuscitation Council

**ANO** (Air Navigation Orders)   These are the regulations and legal framework governing all aspects of flying in and around the UK

**Aramid**   An aromatic polyamide produced by spinning a solid fibre from solution. It is better known by trade names such as Kevlar (DuPont). Aramid is used in the manufacture of lightweight oxygen cylinders and bullet proof jackets

**ARDS** (adult respiratory distress syndrome)   A life-threatening, often fatal, inflammatory disease of the lung characterised by the onset of pulmonary oedema and respiratory failure, in which inflammation of the lungs and accumulation of fluid in the alveoli leads to low blood oxygen levels. There are numerous predisposing conditions such as sepsis, pneumonia and multiple trauma

**ATLS** (Advanced Trauma Life Support)   The ATLS is published by the American College of Surgeons and provides a framework for the management of the injured patient and has its origins in the USA in 1976

**AVPU**   The AVPU scale was developed in the 1980s for the rapid neurological assessment of trauma patients, and stands for Alert, Voice, Pain, Unresponsive

**BP**   Blood pressure

**British Standards**   These are standards that regulate the design and construction of many items in everyday use. Increasingly, these standards are adopted from European standards

**CAA** (Civil Aviation Authority)   A public corporation, established by parliament in 1972 as an independent specialist aviation regulator. The CAA deals with economic regulation, airspace policy, safety regulation and consumer protection. Air traffic control (National Air Traffic Services or NATS) became a separate entity in 2001. See http://www.caa.co.uk

**Capnograph**   The display, or printout, from a capnometer which demonstrates the rising concentration of expired carbon dioxide during expiration of gas from the lung

*Neonatal, Adult and Paediatric Safe Transfer and Retrieval: A Practical Approach to Transfers*, First Edition.
Edited by Bernard Foëx, Peter-Marc Fortune and Cassie Lawn.
© 2019 John Wiley & Sons Ltd. Published 2019 by John Wiley & Sons Ltd.

**Capnometer**    A medical device for measuring expired carbon dioxide, often referred to as a capnography

**CBRN** (chemical, biological, radiological and nuclear)    This describes the risks of accidental spillage, or deliberate release of a variety of toxic materials, and mechanisms for dealing with these spillages

**CCU**    Critical care unit

**CDC** (Communicable Disease Surveillance Centre)    The CDC was founded in 1946 to help control malaria. Its principal role is supporting the US government in protecting the health and safety of Americans, although the CDC is recognised as a worldwide resource in public health efforts to prevent and control infectious and environmental health threats. See http://www.cdc.gov/

**CDR Weekly**    *See* Communicable Disease Report Weekly

**CDSC**    Communicable Disease Surveillance Centre

**CEN**    European Committee for Standardisation

**Children's Act 2004**    UK legislation designed to protect children. Families, healthcare systems and the courts must ascertain and be responsive to the wishes, feelings and physical, emotional and educational needs of children in their care

**CLDP**    Chronic lung disease of prematurity

**CNS**    Central nervous system

**CO**    Cardiac output

**Communicable Disease Report Weekly** (CDR Weekly)    This is the national public health bulletin for England and Wales. Published every Thursday, it has been an exclusively electronic journal since 2001, and has been published as an open circulation bulletin from 1991 onwards. See https://www.gov.uk/health-and-social-care/health-protection-services-health-surveillance-and-reporting-programmes

**Competency based training**    Training for health professionals based upon the participant's ability to demonstrate attainment or mastery of clinical skills to specific standards. The skills are often tasks that require the development of motor functions, although some skills are knowledge and attitude based. When a skill is performed to a specific standard under specific conditions, the skill then becomes a competency. Competencies should be identified and verified in advance. The assessment of competency takes the participant's knowledge and attitudes into account but requires actual performance of the competency as the primary source of evidence. In theory, participants should progress through their educational programme at their own rate, attaining specified competencies as they achieve them

**COPD** (chronic obstructive pulmonary disease)    COPD is now the preferred term for conditions in patients with airflow obstruction who were previously diagnosed as having chronic bronchitis or emphysema. The airflow obstruction is due to a combination of airway and parenchymal damage. The airflow obstruction is usually progressive, not fully reversible, and does not change markedly over several months. Airflow obstruction is defined as a reduced $FEV_1$ (forced expiratory volume in 1 second) and a reduced $FEV_1$/FVC ratio (where FVC is forced vital capacity), such that $FEV_1$ is less than 80% predicted, and $FEV_1$/FVC is less than 0.7. There is no single diagnostic test for COPD. Making a diagnosis relies on clinical judgement based on a combination of history, physical examination and confirmation of the presence of airflow obstruction using spirometry

**CPAP** (continuous positive airways pressure)    CPAP normally describes positive intra-pleural pressure at the end of expiration in the spontaneously breathing patient. Like PEEP (positive end expiratory pressure), the pressure within the lung, even at the end of an expired breath, is never allowed to fall to atmospheric pressure. Both CPAP and PEEP, by preventing distal alveolar collapse, are said to increase the functional residual capacity (FRC) of the lung; this increased FRC acts as an intra-pleural reservoir of oxygenated gas. CPAP is usually delivered using a tight fitting cushioned mask attached to an expiratory pressure regulating valve

**CPP** (cerebral perfusion pressure)    Defined as the difference between the mean arterial blood pressure and the intracranial pressure (MAP – ICP). This calculated number gives a value to the global perfusion pressure of the brain

**CT**    Computerised tomography

**CVP**    Central venous pressure

**CXR**    Chest X-ray

**DC**    Direct current

**DGH**    District general hospital

**DIC**    Diffuse intravascular coagulation

**DKA**    Diabetic ketoacidosis

**DuoDERM**®    One of the Granuflex® families of hydrocolloid dressings. It consists of a flexible, polyurethane outer foam layer and an adhesive skin contact layer which contains a moisture absorbing hydrocolloid material. DuoDERM® is made by Convatec

**EC135**    A lightweight helicopter with a shrouded tail rotor. A common choice by public services, the EC135 is made by Eurocopter in France

**ECG**    Electrocardiogram

**ECMO**    Extracorporeal membrane oxygenation

**ED** (emergency department)    The name used throughout this text to describe an emergency admission facility. The term covers accident and emergency departments (A&Es) and emergency admissions units (EAUs).

**EDV** (end-diastolic volume)    The volume of blood remaining in the cardiac ventricles at the end of filling – the diastole

**Endothelium**    The cellular lining of all blood vessels which is actively involved in the body's inflammatory responses

**ENT**    Ear, nose and throat

**ET tube**    Endotracheal tube

**EtCO$_2$**    End-tidal carbon dioxide

**European pharmacopoeia**    Common name for the European Directorate for the Quality of Medicines (EDQM), which aims to unify manufacturing and quality control standards for pharmaceuticals within the European Union

**European standards**    These are developed by the European Committee for Standardisation or Comité Européen de Normalisation (CEN). This European standards body produces standards covering all aspects of life and industry. After standards are adopted, they are published in each member state by the national standards making organisation (the British Standards Institute (BSI) in the UK). Thus, EN 1795 is published by the BSI as BS EN 1795

**Eurosurveillance**    An organisation that disseminates information to support effective communicable disease surveillance and prevention across Europe. See http://www.eurosurveillance.org/

**FiO$_2$**    Fraction of inspired oxygen

**FRC**    Functional residual capacity

**FS**    Fractional shortening

**GCS** (Glasgow Coma Scale)    The Glasgow Coma Scale (also known as the Glasgow Coma Score or simply GCS) was first published by Teasdale and Jennett in 1974 to assess head trauma referrals to the neurosurgical institute in the Southern General Hospital Glasgow, and, more importantly, to help keep track of patients' progress over a period of time

**HAZIMMS**    Hazardous Materials Incident Medical Management and Support

**HDU**    High dependency unit

**HEMS** (Helicopter Emergency Medical Service)    An air ambulance with a doctor on board, such as the HEMS service based at the London Hospital

**HFOV**    High frequency oscillatory ventilation

**HiB**    *Haemophilus influenzae* type B

**HME**    Humidity and moisture exchanger

**HPA** (Health Protection Agency)    An independent body that plays a critical role in protecting people from infectious diseases and in preventing harm when hazards involving chemicals, poisons or radiation occur. The agency was formed in 2003 and plays an active role in advising about personal protective equipment and preparedness in general. See http://www.hpa.org.uk/

**HR**   Heart rate

**Hypoxaemia**   When the oxygen tension in arterial blood is less than 80 mmHg (10.6 kPa)

**Hypoxia**   A deficiency of oxygen at the tissue level. There are several types:

*Hypoxic hypoxia* in which oxygen tension of arterial blood is reduced   *Anaemic hypoxia* in which the arterial oxygen tension is normal but the amount of haemoglobin (Hb) available to carry oxygen is reduced   *Stagnant or ischaemic hypoxia* in which blood flow to the tissues is so low that oxygen is not delivered to the tissues, despite normal arterial oxygen tension and Hb concentration   *Histotoxic hypoxia* in which oxygen is delivered to the tissues, but a toxic agent prevents the cells using the oxygen

**IABP** (intra-aortic balloon pump)   A two-balloon catheter system inserted via the femoral artery into the thoracic aorta. Sequential inflation of the balloons in time with the cardiac cycle forces blood down the coronary arteries during diastole

**ICBIS** (Intensive Care Bed Information Service)   A comprehensive critical care bed locating service based in the northwest of England. The ICBIS has links into the National ICU Bed Register (NICBR) and supports a local ongoing audit of critical care transfers

**ICP**   Intracranial pressure

**ICS** (Intensive Care Society)   Founded in 1970 to bring together clinicians whose main interest is caring for critically ill patients. Membership includes anaesthetists, surgeons and physicians. The society also has a rapidly growing nurse and professionally allied membership. The society facilitates educational activities and the maintenance of professional standards by liaising with the Royal Colleges of Anaesthetists, Surgeons and Physicians and the Faculty of Intensive Care Medicine. The ICS has continued to improve critical care for patients by working with the Department of Health's Modernisation Agency. See www.ics.ac.uk and www.scottishintensivecare.org.uk/

**ICU**   Intensive care unit

**IO**   Intraosseous

**IV**   Intravenous

**IVH**   Intraventricular haemorrhage

**JRCALC**   Joint Royal Colleges Ambulance Liaison Committee

**Le Fort fracture**   An accepted standard way of describing mid-facial fractures, from the low mid-face Le Fort I fracture, through to the Le Fort III, a total separation of the face from the skull base

**Macrophages**   Tissue monocytes (*see also* Phagocytosis)

**MAP** (mean arterial blood pressure)   The average pressure during the cardiac cycle which is approximately equal to the diastolic pressure (DP) plus one-third of the difference between the DP and systolic pressure (SP):. MAP = DP + 1/3(SP − DP) in mmHg

**MAS**   Meconium aspiration syndrome

**Medical passenger**   The official Civil Aviation Authority designation of a healthcare professional, who has received specified training before being carried in an air ambulance. The minimum training is a pilot briefing around about helicopter safety, specific to the helicopter in use

**MHRA** (Medicines and Healthcare products Regulatory Agency)   The MHRA replaced the Medical Devices Agency (MDA) and the Medicines Control Agency (MCA) in 2003. The regulator's functions are to ensure safety and quality in the supply of medicines and medical devices. See http://www.mhra.gov.uk/

**MOD**   Ministry of Defence

**MRI**   Magnetic resonance imaging

**NAO** (National Audit Office)   The NAO audits the financial statements of all government departments and agencies and many other public bodies. The NAO also reports to parliament on expenditure and value for money

**NEC**   Necrotising enterocolitis

**NHS**   National Health Service

**NiCd**  Nickel cadmium

**NICU**  Neonatal Intensive Care Unit

**NiMH**  Nickel metal hydrate

**NMC** (Nursing and Midwifery Council)  An organisation set up by parliament to protect the public by ensuring that nurses and midwives provide high standards of care to their patients and clients. To achieve its aims, the NMC maintains a register of qualified nurses, midwives and specialist community public health nurses, sets standards for education, practice and conduct, provides advice for nurses and midwives, and considers allegations of misconduct or unfitness to practice due to ill health

**NO**  Nitric oxide

**Oxylog™**  A family of transport ventilators made by Draeger-Medical.

**$PaCO_2$**  Partial pressure of carbon dioxide in alveoli

**Paediatric Intensive Care Society**  This was founded in 1987 as a multi-disciplinary group for those with an interest and involvement in paediatric intensive care. It aims to provide specialist advice, a forum for discussion and also training and education

**PAFC** (pulmonary artery balloon flotation catheter)  The PAFC is also called a right heart catheter or a Swan–Ganz catheter. It is a specialised venous catheter designed to provide information about blood pressures within the heart. The balloon-tipped flotation (Swan) thermodilution (Ganz) catheter passes through the right side of the heart and into the pulmonary artery where the tip lies. The catheter allows measurement of the pulmonary capillary wedge pressure, and the presence of a thermistor near the tip allows calculation of the cardiac output by the Fick principle

**$PaO_2$**  Partial pressure of oxygen in alveoli

**PAPR** (powered air purifying respirator)  A hood or helmet worn as protection against airborne contamination. Air is pumped into the hood through a fine filter

**$pCO_2$**  Partial pressure of carbon dioxide

**PCWP** (pulmonary capillary wedge pressure)  The pressure within the pulmonary vein measured using a pulmonary artery balloon flotation catheter. PCWP is considered as representational of the filling (preload) pressure of the left ventricle

**PEEP** (positive end-expiratory pressure)  A positive intrapleural pressure at the end of expiration that helps to prevent alveolar collapse (*see also* CPAP)

**Personal Protective Equipment Regulations 1992**  These form part of a series of health and safety regulations and replace a number of old and often excessively detailed laws. The effect of the PPE at Work Regulations is to ensure that certain basic duties governing the provision and use of PPE apply to all situations where PPE is required. The regulations follow sound principles for the effective and economical use of PPE, which all employers should follow

**PFC**  Persistent fetal circulation

**Phagocytosis**  A process describing the engulfment and destruction of extracellularly derived materials by phagocytic cells, such as macrophages and neutrophils

**PICANET**  Paediatric Intensive Care Audit Network

**PiCCO**  A device that measures cardiac parameters using transpulmonary thermodilution techniques and arterial pulse contour analysis

**PICU**  Paediatric intensive care unit

**Pneupac**  The name of a company that manufactures a number of different transport ventilators (Transpac™, Parapac™, Ventipac™ and Babypac™). Pneupac is part of Smiths Medical

**Poiseuille's Law**  This describes liquid or gas flows. In laminar flow, the volume of a homogeneous fluid or gas passing per unit time through a capillary tube is directly proportional to the pressure difference between its ends and to the fourth power of its internal radius, and inversely proportional to its length and to the viscosity of the fluid

**PPE** (personal protective equipment) PPE is defined in the PPE regulations as 'all equipment (including clothing affording protection against the weather) which is intended to be worn or held by persons at work and which protects them against one or more risks to their health or safety', e.g. safety helmets, gloves, eye protection, high visibility clothing, safety footwear and safety harnesses. A few types of equipment are not covered by the regulations, mainly ordinary working clothes and uniforms that do not specifically protect against risks to health and safety (*see also* Personal Protective Equipment Regulations 1992)

**PPHN** Persistent pulmonary hypertension of the newborn

**Preload** The volume of blood in the ventricles at the end of diastole

**PTC** Plasma thromboplastin component

**RAF** Royal Air Force

**RDS** Respiratory distress syndrome

**Respirator** A close fitting mask, or hood, designed to give the highest level of protection against airborne contamination of the respiratory tract. The performance of respirators with tight fitting face pieces depends on achieving good contact between the wearer's face and the seal on the mask, something which cannot be assessed by eye or feel. COSHH (Control of Substances Hazardous to Health) Regulations require 'fit testing' to be carried out on respiratory protective equipment (RPE) with tight fitting face pieces

**RIDDOR** (Reporting of Dangerous Occurrences Regulations) This refers to the Reporting of Injuries, Diseases and Dangerous Occurrences Regulations 1995, which came into force in April 1996. RIDDOR requires the reporting of all work-related accidents, diseases and dangerous occurrences

**RNAS** Royal Naval Air Rescue

**RSV** Respiratory syncytial virus

**SaO$_2$** Saturation of oxygen (arterial blood)

**SARS** Severe acute respiratory syndrome

**SCBU** Special care baby unit

**Seldinger guidewire** A generic term used to describe a technique in which a guidewire is passed through a needle; the needle is withdrawn and an intravascular catheter is passed over the guidewire. The technique is commonly used for placing central venous and arterial cannulae; its use has recently been extended to include the passage of a chest drain into the intrapleural space

**SET** Signal extraction technology

**SLA** Sealed lead acid

**Sopite syndrome** A disturbance caused by motion characterised by drowsiness and mood changes that may occur without the classic symptoms of motion sickness; in medical transport personnel, 46% of personnel reported nausea and 65% reported sleepiness caused by motion

**SpO$_2$** Transcutaneous peripheral oxygen saturation

**Surviving Sepsis Campaign** An international campaign aimed at increasing public and healthcare awareness of sepsis, and the promotion of a standardised method for early recognition and treatment. The campaign is supported by the international critical care societies

**SV** (stroke volume) The amount of blood ejected by the ventricle each time it contracts

**SVR** (systemic vascular resistance) This refers to the resistance to blood flow offered by all the systemic vasculature, excluding the pulmonary vasculature. SVR is therefore determined by factors that influence vascular resistance in individual vascular beds. Mechanisms that cause vasoconstriction increase SVR and those that cause vasodilation decrease SVR. Although SVR is primarily determined by changes in blood vessel diameters, changes in blood viscosity also affect it

**SVT** Supraventricular tachycardia

**TcCO$_2$** Transcutaneous carbon dioxide

**TcO₂**  Transcutaneous oxygen

**TPN**  Total parental nutrition

**UAC**  Umbilical arterial catheter

**UVC**  Umbilical venous catheter

**Ventipac™**  A transport ventilator made by Pneupac (Smiths Medical)

**Veress™ laparascopic insufflation needle**  A hollow needle with side holes and a self-retracting stylette. It is used, during some forms of laparoscopic surgery, for the initial abdominal puncture and insufflation of the abdominal cavity with gas

**VQ**  Ventilation/perfusion

**VQ mismatch** (lung ventilation and perfusion mismatch)  This describes a spectrum of abnormalities: at one end alveoli are ventilated but not perfused (pure dead space ventilation); at the other end alveoli are perfused but not ventilated (pure shunt)

**VT**  Ventricular tachycardia

**Waters circuit**  An anaesthetic breathing system classified by the mathematician Mapleson as 'Mapleson C'. Strictly speaking, the original Waters circuit had a soda lime absorber in the circuit. The circuit requires a gas flow (oxygen) as the patient cannot entrain air from outside. Unlike a conventional self-inflating bag–mask–valve, without a gas flow, the Waters circuit cannot be used to hand ventilate a patient

# Index

Page references for glossary entries, figures and tables are given as, for example, 207g, 15f, 24t. Figures and tables are indexed only if there is no other information on that topic on the page.

*Neonatal, Adult and Paediatric Safe Transfer and Retrieval: A Practical Approach to Transfers*, First Edition.
Edited by Bernard Foëx, Peter-Marc Fortune and Cassie Lawn.
© 2019 John Wiley & Sons Ltd. Published 2019 by John Wiley & Sons Ltd.